Principles and Practice of Managing Pain

A Guide for Nurses and Allied Health Professionals

Gareth Parsons and Wayne Preece

Open University Press

Open University Press
McGraw-Hill Education
McGraw-Hill House
Shoppenhangers Road
Maidenhead
Berkshire
England
SL6 2QL

email: enquiries@openup.co.uk
world wide web: www.openup.co.uk

and Two Penn Plaza, New York, NY 10121-2289, USA

First published 2010

A catalogue record of this book is available from the British Library

ISBN-13: 978-0-33-523599-5 (pb)
ISBN-10: 0335235999 (pb)

Library of Congress Cataloging-in-Publication Data
CIP data applied for

Typeset by RefineCatch Limited, Bungay, Suffolk
Printed in the UK by Bell & Bain Ltd, Glasgow

Fictitious names of companies, products, people, characters and/or data that may be used herein (in case studies or in examples) are not intended to represent any real individual, company, product or event.

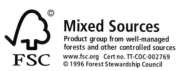

Mixed Sources
Product group from well-managed
forests and other controlled sources
www.fsc.org Cert no. TT-COC-002769
© 1996 Forest Stewardship Council

FSC

The McGraw·Hill Companies

Principles and Practice
of Managing Pain

to be returned on or
last   e below

For Ann, Becca, Tom, Rhodri and Mum

and

For Sue, Aimee, Beth, Nia, Molly, Marc, James and Mam and Dad

Praise for this book

"The recent survey of undergraduate pain education in the UK for health professionals highlights the limited pain education that many receive and makes this a very timely and welcome text. The book is written by experienced pain educators and reflects their wide knowledge and understanding of the key issues in relation to pain and its management which are addressed in the book. The use of a variety of reflective activities as well as clear aims and summaries of the key learning points makes this an excellent resource for health care professionals aiming to become informed carers of those with pain."

Dr Nick Allcock, Associate Professor, University of Nottingham School of Nursing,
Midwifery and Physiotherapy, UK

"I enjoyed reading this book immensely. It is written in an easy to understand style, has a logical progression and contains interesting `real life' scenarios. Each chapter encourages the reader to explore the background issues followed by useful information to assist in an understanding of the complexity surrounding pain and its effective management."

Eileen Mann, Previously Nurse Consultant, Poole Hospital NHS Trust and Lecturer,
Bournemouth University, now retired.

Contents

List of figures   xi
List of tables   xii
About the authors   xiii
Acknowledgements   xiv
Introduction   xv

1. **What is pain?**   1
    Introduction   1
    The importance of defining pain   2
    Classifications of pain   4
    Perspectives on pain   10
    Summary   17
    Reflective activity   17
    References   17

2. **Dilemmas in pain management**   19
    Introduction   19
    Principles   20
    Moral and ethical principles   20
    Effects of illness on moral behaviour   20
    Morals and pain   22
    Deontology   23
    Utilitarianism   25
    Performing a moral calculus   25
    Rights and duties   28
    Bioethics   28
    The best way to organize pain management   33
    Considering the particular nature of pain in developing principles of managing pain   34
    Summary   34
    Reflective activity   35
    References   35
    Further reading   36

3. **Communicating the experience of pain**   37
    Introduction   37
    Intrapersonal perspective of pain   38
    Biopsychosocial model and communication   39
    The intrapersonal nature of pain   40
    Detection and modulation   42
    Cutaneous receptors   42

Contents

Visceral receptors 43
Inflammation and primary hyperalgesia 43
Action potentials 43
Sensory nerve communication 44
The pain gate 44
Ascending pathway 46
The brain 46
Differing pain experiences 48
Interpersonal pain 52
Influences on pain responses 53
The pain experience 55
Something lost in the translation 57
Iatrogenic communication 57
Summary 58
Reflective activity 58
References 59

4. **Pain assessment** 61
Introduction 61
Pain assessment 62
Assessment as part of care planning 63
Problems associated with pain assessment 63
The pain management process 64
Why assess acute pain? 68
Pain assessment tools 70
Pain assessment in children 73
The assessment of chronic pain 75
The character of pain 77
Psychosocial assessment 77
Functional assessment 78
Pain history assessment 78
Questionnaire methods 78
Pain diaries and journals 81
Chronic pain assessment in children 81
Summary 82
Reflective activity 82
References 83
Further reading 85

5. **The pharmacology of pain control** 87
Introduction 87
Mechanisms for drug action 88
Choice of analgesia 88
Drug effectiveness 89
Drug delivery 91
Routes of administration 93
Different routes 93
Plasma concentration 95
Duration of action 96

The three main groups of analgesics 99
Other drugs used in the treatment of pain 105
Summary 107
Reflective activity 107
References 107
Further reading 108

6. **Delivering pain management** 109
   Introduction 109
   The organization of pain management 110
   Development of chronic pain services 110
   The palliative care service 111
   The acute pain service (APS) 111
   Patient education 113
   Risk management 115
   Staff support and development 120
   Summary 121
   Reflective activity 122
   References 122

7. **Acute pain management: planning for pain** 125
   Introduction 125
   The physical effects of unmanaged acute pain 126
   The surgical stress response 127
   Balanced analgesia 128
   Patient-controlled analgesia (PCA) 128
   Person-centred pain management 131
   Ensuring adherence to care 134
   The pain management plan 136
   Summary 139
   Reflective activity 140
   References 141

8. **Chronic pain management** 143
   Introduction 143
   The problem of chronic pain 144
   The prevalence of chronic pain in the UK and Europe 144
   Chronic pain and chronic pain syndrome (CPS) 146
   Specific treatment approaches 149
   The chronic pain management plan 149
   Dealing with pain behaviours 154
   Summary 157
   Reflective activity 158
   References 158

9. **Pain management in palliative care** – *by Maria Parry* 161
   Introduction 161
   Definition of key concepts 162
   Life-limiting conditions 164
   Defining pain in life-limiting conditions 165

Cancer pain   165
Multiple sclerosis (MS) and pain   166
HIV/AIDS and pain   168
Pain assessment   169
Pain assessment tools in palliative care   170
Psychosocial factors influencing the pain experience   171
Barriers to pain assessment and management   174
Pharmacological and non-pharmacological management of pain in palliative care   175
Approaches to pain management in patients who have cancer   175
Drug management   176
The analgesic ladder   177
Immobilization   180
Rehabilitation – modification of daily activities   181
Summary   181
Reflective activity   182
References   182
Further reading   184

Appendix   185
Glossary   187
Index   193

Figures

1.1 Pain in the neck   3
1.2 Normal and abnormal pain   5
1.3 Hierarchy of systems in the biopsychosocial model   13
1.4 The total pain experience   15
3.1 The intrapersonal perspective of pain   39
3.2 Ascent of second-order neurone up the spinothalamic tract   47
3.3 Interpersonal model of pain   53
3.4 Sociocommunication model   55
4.1 The pain management process   65
4.2 Vicious cycle of pain, anxiety and sleeplessness   67
4.3 Example of a pain chart   71
4.4 Visual analogue scale   73
4.5 Numerical graphic rating scale   73
4.6 Wong Baker FACES pain rating scale   74
5.1 A single compartment model of pharmacokinetics   92
5.2 A two compartment model of pharmacokinetics   92
5.3 A three compartment model of pharmacokinetics targeting the central nervous system   93
5.4 Plasma concentration after a single dose of a drug   95
5.5 Repeat dosing before half life reached   97
5.6 Repeat dosing of analgesia at intervals much greater than half life   98
5.7 Pain-free administration of intramuscular morphine   98
5.8 Steady state infusion of intravenous morphine   100
7.1 The principle of balanced or multimodal analgesia   129
7.2 The PCA feedback loop   130
8.1 Duration of chronic pain of intensity 5 or more on a 1–10 NRS intensity scale   145
8.2 The fear-avoidance model of chronic pain   154
8.3 Activity cycling showing pain scores   155
9.1 Examples of possible causes of pain in cancer   166
9.2 Possible causes of pain in MS   167
9.3 Approaches to pain management in cancer patients   176
9.4 WHO (1986) analgesic ladder   177
A.1 Gibbs's (1988) model of reflection   185

Tables

3.1 The physiological response to pain   41
3.2 Properties of different sensory nerves   43
3.3 Properties of neurotransmitters   46
3.4 Common modulation factors after surgery   49
3.5 Examples of types and characteristics of different pain   50
4.1 Criteria for evaluating pain assessment tools   75
4.2 The golden rules of pain assessment   75
4.3 Differences between acute and chronic pain   76
4.4 Comparison of four questionnaires   80–1
5.1 Some examples of altered drug activity   91
5.2 Common routes used by analgesics   93
5.3 Other common factors affecting repeat dosing   99
5.4 Therapeutic actions and side-effects of NSAIDs   100
5.5 Effects of morphine on the gastrointestinal tract   103
6.1 Variations in staffing of chronic pain services   110
6.2 Reasons why an epidural block might fail   118
6.3 Key elements in dealing with organizational issues   120
7.1 Effects of acute pain on body systems   127
7.2 Definition of basic PCA principles   130
7.3 ASA score   133
7.4 A poorly designed care plan   137
7.5 Criteria for writing a care plan   140
8.1 Common chronic pains by site in descending order of prevalence   145
8.2 Chronic pain syndrome symptoms   147
8.3 Extract from a pain diary showing features of activity cycling   156
     Note: In McCracken and Samuel's (2007) study this person would probably be recognized as an
     'extreme cycler'.
9.1 Examples of potentially life-limiting conditions   165
9.2 Clinical staging of HIV disease   168
9.3 Relationship between WHO analgesic ladder steps and numerical rating scale score   178
9.4 Examples of adjuvant drugs used in palliative care   179

About the authors

Gareth Parsons

Gareth Parsons is a Senior Lecturer at the Faculty of Health, Sport and Science at the University of Glamorgan.

Gareth qualified as nurse in 1987; he originally worked in trauma and orthopaedics but in the 1990s moved into pain management. He established two acute pain services and developed a chronic pain service with nurse-led clinics before moving into education. He is the Award leader for the B.Sc. (Hons.) Managing Pain.

Wayne Preece

Wayne Preece is Principal Lecturer (distance education development) at the Faculty of Health, Sport and Science at the University of Glamorgan.

Wayne qualified as a nurse over 30 years ago, initially specializing in mental health and then cardio-respiratory medical nursing. He became a clinical teacher in a medical unit before becoming a lecturer. He has been involved in the development and delivery of a number of distance education programmes including the B.Sc. (Hons.) Managing Pain. Wayne and Gareth both teach on pre- and post-registration nursing and other health care programmes.

Acknowledgements

This book is the end result of many influences, all of which have contributed to its final shape. We would like to thank all those people who have contributed to the development and formation of the ideas behind this book. This is a long list. In recent years it includes our students and colleagues at the University of Glamorgan. Prior to this our many colleagues in our own clinical practices who we have worked with and our past teachers and mentors who moulded our ideas about working with people. We would like to thank Lyn Harris for providing the cartoons that are included in this book. We would like to acknowledge the encouragement and support that our editor Rachel Crookes and her team have given us. A special thank you goes to all the patients who we have had the good fortune to meet in our careers.

Finally, the lion's share of our appreciation falls on our families, our wives, Ann and Sue, our children and grandchildren.

The publisher wishes to acknowledge IIT Bombay (http://www.designofsignage.com/index.html) for allowing permission to use the icon in the case study boxes.

Introduction

Please read me first!

Please read me first! is a phrase that is often included in the instructions for equipment or furniture that has to be assembled. This plea probably recognizes our reluctance to read the preamble and our preference to just jump right in to using the equipment, or putting together the furniture. We have frequently done this, to our cost. While thinking about writing this book, we came to appreciate that we also tended to skip the *Introductions* to books, going straight to the contents or index pages to find the relevant information as quickly as possible. Of course, that may be an appropriate strategy for finding out bits of information but we hope that you will use this book for more than just that purpose. Therefore please *read this introduction first*.

The book is primarily intended as an introduction to pain management for people learning to be an informed carer and so should be of use, for example, to students of nursing, medicine and of professions allied to medicine. We also think it will be of value to those already qualified in those professions.

In writing this book we wanted to achieve two things.

An introductory text

First, we wanted to offer an introductory text to the management of pain. Pain management is the responsibility of all health carers. It does not matter where you specialize or what your interests are, the management of pain will have to find a place in your repertoire of skills. As a result, this book offers chapters covering how pain is defined, some dilemmas associated with pain management, how pain is communicated, and how pain is assessed, managed and evaluated. When considering the management of pain, we offer guidance on acute, chronic and palliative pain care. We have, by necessity, restricted the focus of these discussions to a narrow range of situations; although we are confident that the principles highlighted here can be considered more widely.

Critical reflective practitioners

Second, we hope to encourage you to be a critical reflective practitioner in the management of pain. As a result, you will find within this book activities that will encourage you to engage with the content. Often these are related to your own professional or personal experiences of pain. The activities will also encourage you to be an active reader, rather than a passive scanner of text; something that can occur when reading more traditionally formatted textbooks. This is an approach we have used in developing distance learning material and have found to be very useful in encouraging learning. We have also included a reflective activity at the end of each chapter. These activities take two forms. The first asks you to consider what you have gained from reading the chapter and in so doing encourages critical thought and the content's application to practice. The second form of the reflective activity is through the use of a reflective model. We refer to the one developed by Gibbs (1988) which we have used for some time now within our own practice, learning and teaching. You may already be familiar with other reflective models which you would prefer to use. Reflective practice is considered a means by which we can enhance our personal practice through the thoughtful exploration of real incidents in the light of our present understanding and other forms of evidence.

Decision-making in pain management

All decisions we make about pain management should be based on evidence and, through your critical reflections, we would hope to encourage you to question the evidence on which your practice is based and the practice to which you contribute. We have not been able to include within this textbook a discussion on forms of evidence or a consideration of the decision-making process. When thinking of evidence we often consider this to mean research, but other forms of evidence also exist. Health care has always drawn on a wide range of evidence bases, including the 'medical' and social sciences as well as nursing and midwifery and the many other therapies that contribute to care. When treating our patients/clients we apply evidence from medical and pharmacological research, from communication studies and psychology and sociology, and from studies in management processes. This gives us a broad background, which in turn aids understanding and allows us to assess the individual holistically and offer individualized care. For example, when caring for a patient or client in pain we would have to consider, among many others:

- their ability to communicate;
- their knowledge and understanding of their problem;
- what would be the right treatment or care for that person;
- how receptive they are to any treatments we might offer;
- how to ensure compliance with that treatment;
- how to administer the appropriate care or treatment;
- how to minimize risks and complication.

To achieve this we have to synthesize a wide range of evidence (knowledge) from a variety of sources in order to make effective decisions. As a result, the evidence may come from sources of varying reliability and rigour. This forces us to consider the nature of evidence and our confidence in its validity, applicability and appropriateness.

Developing knowledge

Rycroft-Malone et al. (2004) suggest that knowledge is derived from four sources:

1. research evidence;
2. clinical experience;
3. patients, clients and carers;
4. local context and environment.

It is useful to consider the source of information when reflecting on the evidence that informs your care. There are many very good evidence-based practice and research methodology textbooks available that cover this content. This is an area which needs serious study and we would want to encourage you to gain an understanding of research methodology and other forms of evidence so that you can develop your practice in a dynamic way, as our understanding changes in the light of new evidence.

And finally . . . most of all we want you to enjoy this book. It is one in which you can dip in to find out specific pieces of information, but it can also be used as a programme of study where you can start at the beginning and work your way through.

References

Gibbs G., (1988) *Learning by Doing: A Guide to Teaching and Learning Methods*. Oxford: Further Education Unit, Oxford Polytechnic.

Rycroft-Malone, J., Seers, K., Tirchen, A., Harvey, G., Kitson, A. and McCornmack, B. (2004) What counts as evidence in evidence-based practice? *Journal of Advanced Nursing* 47(1): 81–90.

What is pain?

1

Chapter contents

Introduction
The importance of defining pain
Classifications of pain
Function
Duration
Pathophysiology
Source

Perspectives on pain
The biomedical model
The biopsychosocial model
Summary
Reflective activity
References

Introduction

The purpose of this chapter is to explore what we mean when we use the term 'pain'. This might sound like quite a simple aim but as you will see pain is a complex topic.

Towards the beginning of this chapter we ask you to consider your own experiences of pain. This will form the starting point from which you can compare your present perceptions with the views of others. These initial activities are very important. Do not be tempted to *skip over* them and move on to the theory that follows as throughout this chapter we will be asking you to consider how the opinions of others are consistent, or not, with your view of the pain experience.

There are five broad areas that are covered in this chapter. They are:

(1) the importance of defining pain;
(2) your pain experiences;
(3) classifications of pain;
(4) coming to a definition of pain;
(5) models of health and disease and how they help us understand the pain experience.

As a result the following objectives will be addressed:

- identify and reflect on what pain means to you
- critically explore the subjective nature of pain
- attain an in-depth understanding of pain classifications
- explore definitions of pain
- examine models that give meaning to the individuality of the pain experience
- compare and contrast two models that represent current perspectives on health care.

The importance of defining pain

The usage of individual terms in medicine often varies widely. That need not be a cause of distress provided that each author makes clear precisely how he employs a word. Nevertheless, it is convenient and helpful to others if words can be used which have agreed technical meanings.

(IASP, 2008)

In an ideal situation a clearly detailed definition of pain is important for a number of reasons.

- It allows patients/clients to be open about their experiences of pain.
- It allows carers to communicate with their patients/clients in a way that avoids misunderstanding.
- It provides a framework for identifying factors that shape the patient/client's experience of pain.
- It ensures that all professionals striving to care for those in pain are able to speak to each other in a way that allows understanding and avoids confusion and therefore ensures that the care provided helps the individual in pain.
- It enables the identification of appropriate therapeutic approaches to deal with the described pain.

However, in practice it is not that easy to define pain in such meaningful ways. Partly this is because the word pain can be interpreted in different ways and has many associations.

Activity 1.1

Think of all the different words that can be used to describe pain.
List 20 of these.

You will probably have listed many words, which describe physical aspects of pain, such as aching, burning, soreness or stinging. However, you may also have selected words which imply an emotional component of pain, such as suffering, torment or torture, or a psychological aspect such as distress.

This process of identifying words to describe an experience of pain and then classifying them according to their nature was carried out by Melzack when he developed the McGill Pain Questionnaire (Wall, 1999). Melzack found that 70 words were commonly used to describe pain. Some of these related to describing the stimulus; for example, searing or stabbing; others to the effect on the victim, such as punishing or nauseating. A third group seemed to quantify how much suffering was present – annoying or unbearable for example. Through extensive testing Melzack established that for each person in pain their experience involved at least three dimensions: sensory, **affective** and evaluative.

Think back to activity 1.1 and think how your list compares with some of the terminology suggested above. The McGill Pain Questionnaire is explored later in this book.

Activity 1.2

Now think of the way pain, or similar words are used in our language. What kind of values do we place upon them?

In the everyday use of language, pain and similar words are put to varied uses aside from the obvious one of describing an actual physical symptom of harm through disease or injury. They are frequently used to describe mental suffering; for example, the pain, or hurt, of grief. Pain can also be used to describe putting oneself under pressure to do something with great care; for example, being painstaking or 'taking pains' with something. Such words can also be used to describe taking time to think over a difficult decision – we 'agonize' over a difficult choice. Finally, pain can be used to describe unpleasant characteristics about another; for example, in the phrase 'he's a pain in the neck'.

This widespread use of pain as a descriptor in language reflects the fact that pain is more than a physical symptom; it is also a feeling or emotion and carries a meaning for the individual. This variation of meaning has consequences when dealing with individuals in pain. This is true for many languages other than English and is reflected in the Latin root for pain, *poena* or punishment.

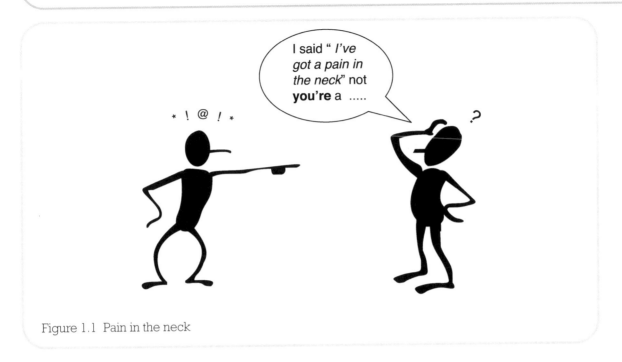

Figure 1.1 Pain in the neck

Our own interpretation of pain may not be the same as our patient's or client's, or indeed, if we were in pain, those caring for us might not understand our pain. This can be a frequent cause of frustration between sufferers and carers.

Most of us have experiences of pain at some time in our life. This may vary from the discomfort associated with mild toothache to more acute pains such as appendicitis or injuries resulting in fracture. It is only in very rare disorders such as congenital insensitivity to pain with anhydrosis (CIPA) that an individual will not have experienced pain. In cases of CIPA people end up harming themselves through normal behaviours, such as eating, because they are unable to sense when too much pressure or biting can cause harm to gums and tongues (Singla et al., 2008).

You may have already had the opportunity to care for patients in pain. The next series of activities in this chapter are going to ask you to explore these personal experiences of pain. Our intent is that you will use these experiences as a starting point for comparison with accepted theory on the nature of pain.

Activity 1.3

Make a list of your experiences of pain. You may like to divide the list into personal experiences of pain, pain experienced by close family or friends and pain experienced by patients in your care.

Activity 1.4

Recall one personal pain experience from your list:

- Try and describe in detail what sensations you experienced and how it made you feel.
- Identify any other factors occurring at the same time which may have contributed to, or detracted from, the degree of pain you experienced.

While you may have found it easy to describe some aspects of the pain; for example, how severe it was and whether it ached or burnt, it might have been quite difficult to describe how the pain made you feel.

Expression of pain can be very difficult within certain cultures. For example, in a study by White (2000) cardiac pain was ignored or denied by a group of men prior to admission to hospital because it does not fit in with their self-image as 'healthy men'. This had serious consequences for this group as they had experienced myocardial infarcts.

Your experiences of pain will be subject to your individual interpretation. However, you may have found that the pain related to an injury while playing a competitive sport was modified by the excitement of the game. On the other hand, a headache experienced when awakening might have felt worse if you knew that a stressful day at work was ahead. In other words context and timing will contribute and alter the meaning of pain.

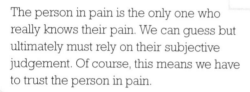

Key point

The person in pain is the only one who really knows their pain. We can guess but ultimately must rely on their subjective judgement. Of course, this means we have to trust the person in pain.

Although we have all experienced pain, it remains a uniquely personal experience. Your experience of toothache will be different from someone else's, for example, although if someone says that they are suffering from toothache you may be able to relate to that experience through memories of your own pain. This variability in pain experience between individuals and in the same individual at different times and under different circumstances would suggest that there are complex mechanisms involved in pain sensation, perception and interpretation. For example, the fact that you are so interested in pain that you are reading this book on the topic may have facilitated your ability to describe your own experiences of pain. Patients and clients who do not have the benefit of your interest, experience and education may find it more difficult to describe and define their pain.

Activity 1.5

Now repeat the last activity, but this time use an example from your list

where pain was experienced by a member of your family, friend or patient.

Try and describe in detail what sensations the individual experienced and how it made them feel.

Identify other factors that occurred at the same time which may have contributed to, or detracted from, the degree of pain experienced.

How easy or difficult did you find it when describing this other person's pain? You may have found that you did not have the same depth of information as you did to recall your own experience. This is understandable. Nevertheless, as health professionals we have to try and understand the other person's perspective and consider factors that may be influencing their pain experience. This is something we return to when examining the assessment of pain later in this book. For now, let us just remind ourselves that individuals may view pain from a different perspective to our own.

This is succinctly illustrated by Bernadette Carter's description of her embarrassment when asking a child to give her a definition of pain:

> When interviewing one 7 year old boy and asking if he could tell me what he thought pain was he looked me straight in the eye sighed heavily and then said: 'Pain hurts – stupid!' This perhaps sums up pain fairly succinctly and reminded me that 7-year olds do not tolerate what they perceive to be daft questions.
>
> (Carter, 1994: 4)

In many instances this would seem to be a fairly straightforward approach to defining pain. However, pain, particularly severe pain, is often an experience that takes over one's mind and body and problems can arise when trying to describe this experience while overpowered by its effects.

Classifications of pain

In order to overcome these problems of defining pain and provide a framework for intervention in and management of pain it is a useful exercise to classify

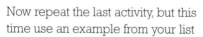

pain. There are several ways this can be done; the commonest ways of classification are by:

- function;
- duration;
- pathophysiology;
- source.

Function

This type of classification depends on looking at pain as a process that normally has a necessary and important function. It has evolved as a strong mechanism to produce aversive or avoiding behaviour to remove an organism from harm or to enable an organism to learn to avoid situations that give rise to pain (Williams, 2002). Where there is an insensitivity to pain; for example, following spinal cord injury, in diabetic neuropathy or in infectious diseases like leprosy (Brand and Yancey, 1994), the protective function of pain is lost and secondary damage often occurs.

For example, the leprosy bacilli *Mycobacterium leprae* damage peripheral nerves in the feet and hands producing a loss of sensation in the peripheral nerves. Paul Brand gives an account of how a man he was treating in India came running to see him on a grossly open fractured and dislocated ankle and did not exhibit any pain despite this injury. He required an amputation to protect him against infection from the dirt he had pushed into his wound when he was running. If this man had suffered a fraction of the pain you or I might imagine experiencing from a dislocated ankle he would have found it painful to hop on crutches, and would have been reluctant to move at all. As it was he ran some distance on his injured ankle causing irreparable damage. In this respect pain can be seen to have a protective function, in which case it is useful and therefore 'normal'. Pain that does not have this function has no protective value and is therefore 'abnormal'. Contrast the experience above with an example you may have experienced, the withdrawing of a finger from a heated surface. In this example of a protective pain reflex you may have noticed that you were withdrawing your finger before perceiving the pain.

Normal pains are those which draw attention to a problem in the body so that we can take suitable action. They protect us because we become aware of the pain, will rest the injured area, will seek help if necessary and will take appropriate actions to prevent a problem getting worse (see Fig. 1.2). They act as a

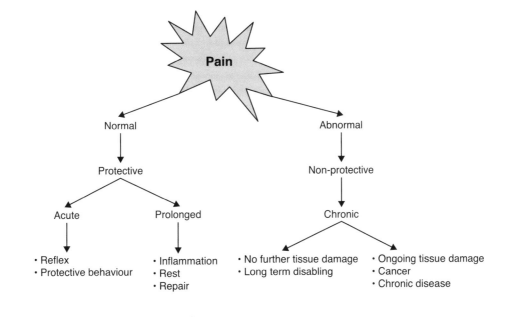

Figure 1.2 Normal and abnormal pain
Source: adapted from Gebhart (2000)

warning that tissue damage is about to occur or as an alarm that tissue damage has occurred. Abnormal pains are those which persist after the initial warning phase, occur where there is no apparent tissue damage or tissue damage has healed or accompany progressive diseases that cannot be cured.

The idea that pain can be classified as normal or abnormal is attractive. It enables us to identify pains that are likely to eventually resolve themselves, 'normal pains' and those that will not. However, it has limitations. If we only rely on this as our way of classifying pain what we are saying is that pain is part of a disease process rather than an illness process; That is, it is a symptom of tissue damage and behavioural and other factors are secondary to this.

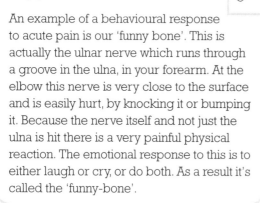

Key point

An example of a behavioural response to acute pain is our 'funny bone'. This is actually the ulnar nerve which runs through a groove in the ulna, in your forearm. At the elbow this nerve is very close to the surface and is easily hurt, by knocking it or bumping it. Because the nerve itself and not just the ulna is hit there is a very painful physical reaction. The emotional response to this is to either laugh or cry, or do both. As a result it's called the 'funny-bone'.

A consequence of this is that we view acute pains as normal, and with most acute pains we know the cause – it might be surgery, toothache or a hangover. Acute pain produces particular behavioural responses in an individual. We know that treating the acute pain, with analgesia for example, will usually reduce this behavioural response. However, if it does not is the pain still normal? For example, if a patient has a much larger dose of analgesia for their acute pain than would usually be given and this has not eased their pain is their pain still normal or is it now abnormal? After all it does not follow the normal pattern of events. This could lead us to regard unusual behaviours displayed during acute pain as abnormal when in fact they are that individual's way of expressing their pain.

Another problem with regarding pain that no longer serves a function as abnormal is that this is not really a satisfactory explanation of the ongoing pathology in some chronic diseases and cancers. For example rheumatoid arthritis produces pain through an ongoing inflammatory process that causes the nervous system to respond in a similar way to toothache. A metastatic spread of cancer will probably induce pain in new structures in just the same way as the pain that first warned us of the onset of cancer. The nervous system is stimulated in the same way as in acute pain, but this stimulation is ongoing.

Duration

A different way of classifying pain is to think about it in terms of its duration. This has been described as '*the most important dichotomy in the pain world*' (Loeser, 2002).

According to this classification pain is either acute or chronic. Acute pain has the following characteristics:

- It is usually a result of tissue injury that has occurred in the very recent past.
- The site of injury is easily detected.

(Loeser, 2002)

- Its intensity and effects subside as healing progresses.
- Its duration is brief from seconds to months at the most.

(McCaffrey and Beebe, 1999)

Even this description is broad because it captures the fleeting pain of a needle-stick injury as well as the aching pain of a fracture or the pain following recovery from surgery. It is therefore important to remember that acute pain does not mean severe pain. A sore throat is an acute pain in the same way that childbirth is an acute pain. Both meet the above criteria.

Chronic pain by contrast has these characteristics:

- The cause of the pain may not be apparent.

This may be because:

- Healing has occurred and the pain is still present.
- Or there is often a question of whether there ever was an injury.

(Loeser, 2002)

- It has lasted for longer than an acute pain would.

Some definitions suggest over three months and others over six months.

- The pain persists and/or worsens with the progress of time.

There are difficulties with using these descriptions of acute and chronic pain, however, as they do not adequately cover pains seen in conditions like migraine. Here the sufferer is usually pain free. When they have pain it is acute, has a limited duration, but is recurrent, sometimes on a weekly basis. It also has limitations when considering ongoing pains which are time limited. McCaffrey and Beebe (1999) suggest that a definition of chronic pain does not adequately describe cancer pain or burn pain. Although the pain occurs daily over a long period it can usually be well controlled by analgesia or other pain-relieving medication. It may last for many months, even years before the condition is cured or controlled or the likelihood of pain may end with death.

Chronic pain therefore means pain that is:

- Difficult if not impossible to control using conventional therapies.
- Is not life ending but is life limiting (that is it is due to non-life threatening causes but has a profound debilitating effect on the individual.)
- May last for the whole of the individual's life – this may be many decades.
- Regardless of the underlying cause, psychological, social and environmental factors will play a significant role in the nature of the pain.

(Loeser, 2002).

Pathophysiology

The third way to look at pain is from its pathophysiology. This can be very useful when considering a therapeutic approach to its management. The two main categories here are nociceptive pain and neuropathic pain.

Nociceptive pain (also written as nocioceptive) essentially describes pain that occurs in a healthy sensory nervous system. That is, the nervous system is not damaged and the pain arises outside of the central nervous system, the brain and the spinal cord, is detected by nerve receptors and transmitted via sensory neurons to the spinal cord and brain. Examples of nociceptive pain include that seen following incisions, such as after surgery or a laceration, or pain following trauma, such as a fractured wrist or dislocated shoulder. These are examples of acute pains but chronic pains can also be nociceptive; a good example is osteoarthritis.

Neuropathic pain refers to pain where the nervous system is compromised in some way. They are also called neurogenic pain because the pain originates in the nervous system. In these pains there may be physical damage to sensory nerves in the periphery; for example, post-herpetic neuralgia, to the spinal nerves, in some low back pains for example, to the spinal cord or to the brain, following a stroke. Damage to the central nervous system is also called central pain.

There may also be physiological changes to an apparently healthy central nervous system as a result of sustained and/or severe nociceptive pain. Such an effect contributes to the phenomenon of phantom limb pain.

Neuropathic pains are characterized by unusual sensations and the pain may feel that it originates in a different part of the body. For example, sciatica is a pain caused by damage to or stretching or compression of the sciatic nerve; this may occur due to a vertebral disc lesion or because of lower back muscle spasm. However, sufferers generally complain of shooting pains radiating downward from the buttock over the posterior or lateral side of the lower limb.

Neuropathic pains do not respond to treatments for nociceptive pain and are often associated with intense emotional suffering. Both nociceptive and neuropathic pain types are seen in acute and chronic pain. Of course, one has to be able to identify the type of pain in order to treat it. Generally, nociceptive pains are viewed as opioid sensitive and neuropathic pains as opioid resistant. That is, nociceptive pains are more likely to respond to drugs such as morphine while neuropathic pains are not. It is worth remembering though that there are many pain syndromes of uncertain or unknown aetiology; for example, the cause of back pain is certain in only a fifth of cases (Loeser, 2002).

Source

The origin of the pain is also used to classify types of pain. This includes neuropathic pains which originate in the nervous system but also includes categories of nociceptive pain and cancer pain.

Cancer pain

Pain in cancer comes from a variety of sources, nociceptive and neuropathic; it may also arise as a result of therapy and there may be multiple pain problems (Simpson, 2000). Although cancer pain has many of the characteristics of chronic pain, in that it may last a long time and affects quality of life for the individual as well as their family, it is worth considering as a special case because of its other characteristics especially in the terminally ill.

Somatic pain

Somatic pain refers to nociceptive pain mainly originating from the skin or skeletal muscle system, muscles, bones, tendons, and so on. It also arises from some deeper structures like the peritoneum. Somatic pain is the most common type of nociceptive pain experienced. It has certain characteristics because it possesses millions of pain-specific receptors and has associated neurones dedicated to these receptors. These characteristics are:

- sensations can be localized easily;
- pain is often intense, may be rapid;
- is carried on myelinated and unmyelinated neurones;
- is caused by trauma or damage to the tissues surrounding the receptors.

Visceral pain

The term 'viscera' refers to the large internal organs of the body. Visceral pain is more diffuse and results from stimulation of non-specific receptors belonging to unmyelinated autonomic nerves that supply organs and other tissues in deeper structures; for example, capsular tissue around internal organs. The stimuli that produce the pain are different. Instead of direct trauma inducing pain it may be produced by distension of hollow organs, like the intestines or stretching of the capsule around solid organs such as the liver. It may also be caused by chemical changes as a result of ischaemia in the viscera, as seen in angina.

The pain is characterized as poorly localized, diffuse cramping or colicky. The pain is often referred to more superficial structures at some distance from the tissue producing the stimuli. In abdominal pain the pain is perceived in the abdominal region that originated from the same embryonic tissue as the damaged viscera. This site might display excessive sensitivity to unpleasant stimuli which is interpreted as pain (hyperalgesia) even though the underlying tissue is undamaged. A characteristic of acute appendicitis is sensitivity to touch around the umbilicus. If diseased, the afflicted viscera may also become hyperalgesic (McMahon, 1997). As a result rectal examination in appendicitis may produce severe pain.

Activity 1.6

Clarify the similarities and differences between cancer pain, somatic pain and visceral pain in relationship to the following characteristics by completing this activity.

	Cancer pain	Somatic pain	Visceral pain
Localized or not			
Stimuli that produce pain			
Nociceptive or neuropathic or both			

A definition of pain

The discussion so far illustrates the complexity of classifying pain. As you can see it is very difficult to come up with a particular definition of pain. The International Association for the Study of Pain (IASP) has attempted to incorporate many of the concepts we have discussed in its definition. *'Pain: An unpleasant sensory and emotional experience associated with actual or potential tissue damage, or described in terms of such damage'* (IASP, 2008).

Activity 1.7

Consider the IASP definition of pain. Do you feel this is a fair summary or could it be further improved? How would you change or add to it?

The IASP qualify their definition with the following remarks. Do they address your concerns?

> *Pain: An unpleasant sensory and emotional experience associated with actual or potential tissue damage, or described in terms of such damage.*
>
> *Note: The inability to communicate in no way negates the possibility that an individual is experiencing pain and is in need of appropriate pain relieving treatment.*
>
> *Notes: Pain is always subjective. Each individual learns the application of the word through experiences related to injury in early life. Biologists recognize that those stimuli which cause pain are liable to damage tissue. Accordingly, pain is that experience we associate with actual or potential tissue damage. It is unquestionably a sensation in a part or parts of the body, but it is also always unpleasant and therefore also an emotional experience.*
>
> *Experiences which resemble pain but are not unpleasant, e.g., pricking, should not be called pain. Unpleasant abnormal experiences (dysaesthesias) may also be pain but are not necessarily so because, subjectively, they may not have the usual sensory qualities of pain.*

Many people report pain in the absence of tissue damage or any likely pathophysiological cause; usually this happens for psychological reasons. There is usually no way to distinguish their experience from that due to tissue damage if we take the subjective report. If they regard their experience as pain and if they report it in the same ways as pain caused by tissue damage, it should be accepted as pain.

(IASP, 2008)

For a fuller description of pain terminologies visit the IASP website at www.iasp-pain.org

Another way of looking at pain is to regard the individual suffering the pain as the expert in their pain. This is an approach first advocated by Margo McCaffrey in 1968, and her definition of pain provides a useful philosophy for pain management. *'Pain is whatever the experiencing person says it is and exists whenever he says it does'* (McCaffrey and Beebe, 1999: 16).

As with the IASP definition McCaffrey has further clarified the underlying principle of this statement with regard to the management of pain.

> *Specifically this definition means that when the patient indicates he has pain, the health team responds positively. The patient's report of pain is either believed or given the benefit of the doubt. Each health team member is entitled to his or her personal opinion about whether the person is telling the truth about his pain. However, the issue is professional responsibility, which is to accept the patient's report of pain and to help the patient in a responsive and positive manner.*

(McCaffrey and Beebe, 1999: 16)

Both these definitions recognize that pain is complex and because it is subjective it can often be difficult to understand and manage. The way the individual reacts to their pain affects the way we interpret what is going on. This is a difficult process and full of pitfalls as you will see as you progress through this book.

Perspectives on pain

Definitions seek to encapsulate the pain experience. This is not a straightforward process. In this section of the chapter we are going to look at different perspectives on health and disease and explore how these can help us come to a more complete understanding of pain and therefore appreciate some of its complexities. Although there are many models available to support practitioners in their understanding of health care we will explore two of the most influential models. These are the biomedical model and the biopsychosocial model.

A model is a description or analogy used to help visualize something in order to help us understand it. A model is used to explain behaviour, assess problems, predict outcomes, organize solutions and enable communication between those who use the model and recognize changes in the situation. A 'good' model while only being a characterization of the object or problem it represents should in practical terms enable the person who uses it to find a workable way of understanding the object or problem and also provide solutions to the problem. Models are therefore not right or wrong and they vary in their ability to account for what is going on.

The biomedical model

In health care the biomedical model has been the dominant framework for explaining disease processes. It is a robust model and is very good at explaining fully or partially many health problems. The biomedical model is successful because it is based on the following principles:

- Linear causality, that is, disease is caused by something.
- It views the body as a biological entity which either functions smoothly – and is therefore healthy or is malfunctioning because of some causative factor – and is therefore diseased.
- It is reductionist. It attempts to explain the biological processes of the body by the same explanations (through physical laws) that chemists and physicists use to interpret inanimate matter.

This provides the biomedical model with some strong tools for identifying and treating health problems as it enables the identification of:

- disease pathogens – for example, leprosy, as we have seen, can be caused by the bacterium *Mycobacterium leprae*;
- disease pathology – for example, diabetes mellitus, which gives rise to a form of neuropathy, is caused by a loss of or inadequate production of insulin by the islets of Langerhans in the pancreas;
- disease patterns – people who drink water from a contaminated source may contract cholera.

This is a very suitable approach for dealing with many health problems as it establishes the causal agents and this knowledge can be used to eliminate the causes of the disease or reduce damage. For this reason the biomedical approach continues to be widely and extensively used as an aid to diagnosis and treatment.

This model's premise is that *'health and disease are considered distinct entities defined by the absence or presence of a specific biological factor'* (Deep, 1999: 496).

The type of approach utilized by the biomedical model is based upon 'factor analysis'. A patient presents with some symptoms and the clinician needs to process these in order to make a diagnosis (usually a doctor although all health professionals acquire and practise these skills). This might involve asking questions to elicit more information, investigating the presence of associated physical signs, arranging for specific tests to be performed. Once all the information is in hand the clinician would then hope to be able to identify a treatable pathology and prescribe a treatment in anticipation of effecting a cure (Cockerham, 2007).

Imagine you are a family doctor and a patient complains to you of feeling woozy. How are you going to establish a cause for this? After all wooziness is not an exact description of a symptom.

You might have a suspicion as to a cause for this strange symptom but you might equally not have an idea. A useful first approach would be to try and establish the exact nature of this woozy feeling. Therefore you might ask some questions, such as what time of day did this occur? What activity were you doing at the time? What was your alcohol consumption? You might also perform some physical tests, a neurological examination, blood pressure and pulse, blood glucose and might arrange for other tests to be carried out, blood samples, and electro-cardiograph, and so on.

Once you have all these facts to hand you then proceed to eliminate causes. Did they feel woozy after getting out of a chair quickly? If not it is probably not postural hypotension. Did they drink a lot of alcohol the night before? Maybe they are still feeling the effects of this. Was their blood pressure high or low? Do they have an unusual electrocardiograph tracing? Then they might have a cardiovascular problem.

Eventually you will come to a diagnosis that says with some certainty that a particular disease process caused this person's symptoms and a treatment programme can be started.

In its purest form this factor analysis relies on reducing any information obtained to physical terms; this can mean that psychological and social data may have little or no influence on diagnosing the problem and may even be seen as getting in the way of finding out what is wrong.

Because many health professionals are educated in this system or work in an environment that is organized around this system, it influences the way practitioners approach patients and clients (Cockerham, 2007). Practitioners are often unaware of the influence the biomedical model has on their practice and education. Additionally, many patients and clients are used to and indeed expect health professionals to act within this framework and this can also be a source of problems as they seek an answer to a problem they have. This can be particularly true where no immediately obvious physical cause for their problem is present or they object to, or do not respond to, or comply with, the prescribed care. A situation that is common in many pain conditions.

Problems with the biomedical model

In practice psychological and social factors are influential in deciding diagnosis and treatment plans although not always in the most helpful way. For example, assessment and management of patients and clients who demonstrate behaviours such as high utilization of time and resources, multiple complaints of symptoms with no apparent cause, anger, non-compliance and anxiety, may evoke a frustrated response from the practitioners as they are unable to satisfy their needs. These patients will be considered difficult and may evoke hostility, avoidance and rejection. This is a source of many complaints about care as patients and clients feel they are not addressed as a whole person. This is particularly true when an individual's behaviour does not match their apparent symptoms.

Activity 1.8

We have covered a number of important concepts related to the biomedical model. It is worth while pausing and writing a response to the following questions to reflect on the material covered so far.

■ Does having a disease mean you are not healthy?

■ Can you feel ill and not have a disease?

■ Are disease and illness the same thing?

These questions may seem a bit odd on first examination – it would seem to be fairly obvious that 'health is good' and 'disease is bad'. In fact, such simple definitions do not often fit with reality because of the highly subjective nature of disease to an individual. As with a definition of pain, a definition of health is also difficult to write and the World Health Organization proposition reflects this: *'Health is a complete state of physical, mental and social well-being and not merely the absence of disease'* (World Health Organization, 1980: 2).

Is it possible to have a disease and be healthy? There are many instances where this may be the case. For example, is someone who has diabetes mellitus unhealthy? If their diabetes is well controlled and they experienced no symptoms as a result then they would probably describe themselves as healthy and would even become upset if they were described as diseased. A different example can be seen in disability: it would be hard to argue that Tanni Grey-Thomson, winner of four wheelchair gold medals in the 2000 Paralympics and two in the 2004 games is unhealthy. In her whole career she has won 16 Paralympic medals, 11 of them gold, has held more than 30 world records, and is six times winner of the London Marathon. A third example may be those who have an underlying disease that has not manifested itself as an illness and shows no apparent symptoms; for example, undiagnosed hypertension.

Is it possible to have an illness and not have a disease? This an area of great controversy because according to the biomedical model there must be some disease process present if one feels ill. This poses big problems for people who fail to have a particular disease identified by a doctor. A common example of this is back pain. This is a major cause of illness in the UK but often no physical site for the pain is identified. Equally controversial perhaps is the effect on an individual when a cure for the disease leaves them feeling ill. Another illustration of this point might be pregnancy. This is not a pathological state but many women experience illness during their pregnancy.

Are disease and illness the same thing? If we accept that people can feel ill without having a bodily cause for this illness then we have to accept that illness and disease are not the same. From a biomedical point of view illness is not a physical process but a social construct.

A common criticism of the biomedical model is that it focuses purely on disease and disease processes and not on the individual although Main and Spanswick (2000) suggest that it works well for most acute medical and surgical conditions. That is, it separates the mind from the body and concentrates solely on the latter. Supporters of the biomedical model have argued that this occurs because not enough is known about how the brain works and a detailed understanding of neurobiology in the future will help to explain many aspects of illness we do not yet understand. This

is quite likely to be so but it does leave health professionals and patients and clients struggling to come to terms with how to deal with our present understanding.

In summary the three key principles of the biomedical model are:

1. All diseases can be explained by disturbances in physiological processes, resulting from, for example injury, biochemical imbalances or the action of a pathogen.
2. Disease is an affliction of the body and is separate from psychological and social processes of mind.
3. Health and disease are separate and incompatible.

The biopsychosocial model

The biopsychosocial model provides a more convenient method for looking at pain in a manner that allows explanation of the complexity and diversity of this phenomenon.

The biopsychosocial model was first proposed by George Engel in 1977 as an alternative framework for looking at those health problems that the existing and well-established biomedical model was unable to solve or completely explain. Engel (1977) worked as a psychiatrist and was frustrated by the fact that the biomedical model that formed the foundation of his training and practice did not fully explain the clinical features presented by his clients.

This model is based on a systems biology approach to health. This is often represented as a hierarchical continuum organized into different levels that overlie each other (see Fig. 1.3).

In this model, instead of the individual being a body that disease works on, the 'person' is centrally placed among the layers and it is recognized that an individual's health may be affected as much by social and other factors external to the body as to processes occurring within it (Fava and Sonino, 2008).

This model addresses many of the problems identified in the biomedical model while allowing the useful aspects of the biomedical model to be retained. Thus, a biopsychosocial approach may be used to identify potential factors in a disease as illustrated by Deep (1999):

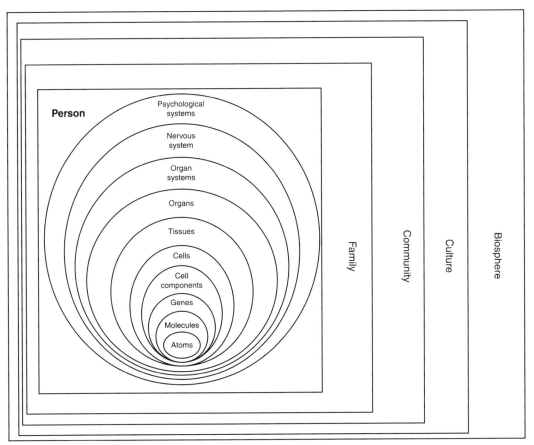

Figure 1.3 Hierarchy of systems in the biopsychosocial model

The oral cavity in most humans is colonized by Streptococcus mutans, *one of the bacteria primarily responsible for caries formation. However not all individuals develop caries. The mere presence of a specific biological factor is not always sufficient to cause disease, which suggests that the biomedical model is inadequate in its scope.*

(Deep, 1999: 496)

So other factors must also be considered before we arise at an understanding as to why an individual may have dental caries.

To illustrate the complexity of the disease processes consider the following activity.

Activity 1.9

Under the following categories identify biopsychosocial reasons for dental caries to form in an individual:

Biological   Behavioural

Emotional   Physical environment

Mental   Social environment

Compare your response with our suggestions below.

- Biological factors: although we have identified the presence of a pathogen, are there other factors to consider? Among others you might have listed: diet, high sugar content drinks, previous decay or injury to teeth. Another physical illness that restricts ability to brush teeth; for example, rheumatoid arthritis.
- Emotional factors you might have considered are anxiety and stress. We might choose to eat more sugary foods and drinks when feeling stressed.
- Mental factors might include personality, intelligence, knowledge of dental hygiene, beliefs about the need to brush or floss teeth, perceptions of risk to disease. Do they avoid the dentist? If they have dental pain do they self-medicate or seek help? Self-esteem. Do they take a pride in their appearance?
- Behavioural factors could include whether they brush their teeth or not, and how often they do it; eating sweets and drinking carbonated cola; attending regular dental checkups and so on.
- Physical environment might include the type of dental cleaning products they use, access to dental care, surgery times, availability of money to pay for care or dental hygiene products, means of transportation, access to shops.

- Social factors might include a family attitude to dental hygiene, education, their relationship with their dentist, whether there is state provision of dental services or whether it is privately financed, attitudes among peers and within their cultural environment to foods and dental hygiene.

You can see from this list that an apparently simple disease like dental caries has many factors that can influence its outcome.

In summary, the biopsychosocial model thinks of the individual as consisting of both biological and psychological systems that interact with each other to make the person. This person exists within a social system and is acted on by this social system while also exerting an influence on the social system.

In pain this concept has been developed to explain the complexity of the pain experience. In some ways it enables the individuality of a person's pain to be identified. Figure 1.4 represents the interaction between the three systems. We can see that there is a degree of overlap between each system and also that all three overlap in the middle. This overlapping segment represents the total pain experience (Saunders, 1984).

This model asserts that pain is much more than a reflection of underlying biological factors, such as extent of injury (Mehta and Chan, 2008). It is also a consequence of psychological phenomena, such as

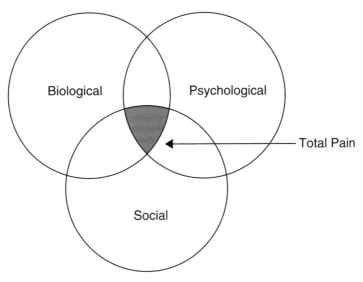

Figure 1.4 The total pain experience
Source: Welsh Health Planning Forum (1992)

mood or learning and social influences; for example, carer's responses (Sutton et al., 2002).

> In a typical month, a normal, otherwise-healthy child averages about 4 acute pains related to injuries and diseases – falls, sore throats, sprains – plus one achy pain, such as a headache or stomach ache. Pain diaries kept by children show a diverse list of pain-causing experiences: being hit on the head with a golf club, stung by a bee, bitten by a dog, stepping on broken glass.
>
> (McGrath, 1998)

Activity 1.10

The quotation from McGrath (1998) indicates what a common experience pain is. However, as we have discussed, our responses to similar physical pains can vary greatly depending on psychological and social factors.

Using the two following examples of acute pain in a child aged 7 discuss why his total pain experiences are different. You may wish to look at Fig. 1.4 when answering these questions.

(1) Mark Walker is playing football in the school playground. He has just scored a goal and is very excited. He is knocked to the ground while tackling to get the ball, bangs his head on the tarmac and sustains a large graze along his knee. His friends laugh at him and he soon gets up and is chasing after the ball again. Later, in class, his teacher asks him if he is all right and Mark says he is fine.

(2) Mark is at home. It is raining and he and his older brother Jason, aged 12, are bored. What starts off as mild name-calling soon becomes a rough and tumble fight and Mark comes off worse. He knocks his head on the wall and grazes his knee on the floor. Mark's mother, Christine, is trying to cook dinner and shouts at Jason when Mark comes into the kitchen crying and complaining of pain. Christine had just told the boys to stop fighting.

Although Mark Walker has sustained very similar injuries in both examples, his responses to them are very different. It would seem reasonable to assume that a head injury and a large graze to the knee would produce a moderate degree of discomfort and pain in both instances. This is what a biomedical approach would do. Yet in our first example Mark does not seem to be in any pain or discomfort, while in the second he appears quite distressed and would probably complain of moderately severe pain.

If however we view the two incidents from a biopsychosocial perspective, we can offer the following explanations of the differing total pain experiences:

- Biologically the two injuries are similar and we would imagine that similar pain messages must have travelled from the sites of injury along Mark's nervous system. However, something must be happening to these messages to produce different perceptions of pain. Perhaps there are other physiological and neurological processes in play. Although both injuries are sustained during physical activity, playing football and fighting with his brother, the nature of the activity is still different. Mark is obviously quite good at football and is enjoying himself whereas a fight with an older brother probably does not bring him as much pleasure and this may produce a stronger pain response. In the first scenario Mark is in a state of arousal, he is exhilarated after scoring a goal, in the second he is bored.

- Psychologically, Mark's obvious pleasure from playing football would provide a distraction from any discomfort. He is enjoying himself and wants to continue to do so. There are also issues of self-esteem and control. Peer pressure and gender expectations may also play a part in appearing stoical. In the second example however Mark may feel less in control of the situation. He might well be used to losing fights with his brother and this will affect his self-esteem. With his mother, gender issues may not be as relevant and as the younger sibling he might not be expected to be as brave as he is among his friends. His normal response to a fight with his brother might be to cry when he is losing and appeal to a parent to exert some control.

- Socially, in the first example, Mark has to maintain his status among his peers. He probably has a reasonably high status as boys of this age admire physical ability (such as scoring goals), he therefore would not wish to appear a 'cry baby'. He is at an age when friends and peers are becoming important shapers of his social behaviour. This would be especially true in the classroom where he can prove his status by brushing off concerns from his teacher. At home however Mark's status is still that of a younger child; this may cause Mark frustrations at times but also allows him to exhibit childish behaviour, such as crying and appealing for help from an adult without social sanction.

We can therefore see how from a biological, psychological and social perspective a similar injury in the same child can produce a markedly different response depending on factors entirely unrelated to the cause of the tissue damage. In this instance a biomedical approach would be insufficient to explain why there is a difference in Mark's pain experience.

Activity 1.11

Now return to the experiences you recalled in Activities 1.4 and 1.5.

How would you classify these events in relation to:

function;
duration;
pathophysiology;
source?

How well did you document these factors during the activities?

Had you fully considered the psychosocial factors during the activities?

This penultimate activity encouraged you to examine your initial documentation of pain experiences in the light of what you have studied during the chapter. Hopefully, the series of activities would have helped you consider the personal nature of pain and its complexity in terms of how the experience is interpreted.

Summary

This chapter has concerned itself with defining pain. In the process you have explored what pain means to you and hopefully you have recognized that pain is a complex phenomenon that is often not easily understood and may be open to misinterpretation. As new understandings of pain have led us to view pain as an illness we recognize that understanding a patient's pain behaviour, thoughts and feelings is just as crucial to managing pain as having knowledge of the physiology of pain and analgesics (Main and Spanswick, 2000).

The main ideas we wished to communicate in this chapter are:

- It is important to recognize your own experiences of pain and pain management.
- A clear definition of pain is important.
- We use a range of words to explain our physical, emotional and social experience of pain.
- Pain can be classified in terms of function, duration, pathophysiology and source. There are strengths and limitations to these classifications.
- Only the individual in pain really knows their pain.
- The pain experience needs to be considered in the wider context of health and disease.
- Biomedical and biopsychosocial models of health and disease help us come to a more complete understanding of pain.
- The biopsychosocial model of health and disease is our preferred model for explaining the complexity and diversity of the pain experience.
- The biopsychosocial model helps us to understand the total pain experience.

Reflective activity

As a conclusion to this chapter consider how knowledge of this theory will help you in your future practice. Try to be specific and use the following points/questions as a guide.

- *State* which elements of the chapter will help you in your future practice.
- *Elaborate:* be specific in terms of how this knowledge and understanding can be used in practice.
- *Give examples* of care events which would benefit from what you have learnt.
- What are the *implications* if you change the way you practise.

You may prefer to use a reflective model such as Gibbs's (1988) to guide your reflection. The model is reproduced in the Appendix at the end of this book. Think of a specific example as the starting point. This may have been included in your list (Activity 1.4). Describe the event and then proceed through the cycle. When analysing the situation draw on this chapter's theory to support your discussion and demonstrate your understanding.

References

Brand, P. and Yancey, P. (1994) *Pain: The Gift Nobody Wants.* London: Marshall Pickering.

Carter, B. (1994) *Child and Infant Pain: Principles of Nursing Care and Management* (Chapter 1). London: Chapman & Hall.

Cockerham, W. C. (2007) *Social Causes of Health and Disease.* Cambridge: Polity Press.

Deep, P. (1999) Biological and biopsychosocial models of health and disease in dentistry, *Journal of the Canadian Dental Association,* 65(9): 496–7.

Engel, G. (1977) The need for a new medical model: a challenge for biomedicine, *Science,* 196(4286): 129–36.

Fava, G.A. and Sonino, N. (2008) The biopsychosocial model thirty years later, *Psychotherapy and Psychosomatics,* 77(1): 1–2.

Gebhart, G.F. (2000) *Scientific issues of pain and distress.* (pp. 22–30) Paper presented at the 'Definition of pain and distress and reporting requirements for laboratory animals': proceedings of the Workshop, Washington, DC on 22, June 2000, Institute for Laboratory Animal Research (ILAR), The National Academies Press Available online at www.nap.edu/openbook.php?record_ id=10035&page=22 (accessed 27 May 2009).

Gibbs G (1988) *Learning by Doing: A Guide to Teaching and Learning Methods.* Oxford: Further Education Unit, Oxford Polytechnic.

International Association for the Study of Pain (2008) IASP pain terminology. Available online at www.iasp-pain.org/ AM/Template.cfm?Section=General_Resource_ Links&Template=/ CM/HTMLDisplay.cfm&ContentID= 3058 (accessed 25 June 2008).

Loeser, J.D. (2002) Pain: Concepts and management: WFSA distance learning. Available online at www.nda.ox.ac.uk/ wfsa/dl/html/ papers/pap024.htm (accessed 19 November 2002).

Main, C.J. and Spanswick, C.J. (2000) *Pain Management: An Interdisciplinary Approach.* London: Churchill Livingstone.

McCaffery, M. and Beebe, A. (1999) *Pain: Clinical Manual,* 2nd edn. St Louis: The C.V. Mosby Company.

McGrath, P. (1998) *Children's pain perception: impact of gender and age.* Paper presented at the *Gender and Pain Conference,* Scientific Abstracts National Institutes of Health Available online at www.painconsortium.nih.gov/ genderandpain/ children.htm (accessed 15 June 2009).

McMahon, S.B. (1997) Are there fundamental differences in the peripheral mechanisms of visceral and somatic pain? *Behavioral and Brain Sciences,* 20(3): 381–91.

Mehta, A. and Chan, L.S. (2008) Understanding of the concept of 'total pain': a prerequisite for pain control, *Journal of Hospice and Palliative Nursing,* 10(1) 26–32.

Saunders, C. (1984) (ed.) *The Management of Malignant Disease,* 2nd edn. London: Arnold.

Simpson, K.H. (2000), Philosophy of cancer pain management, in K.H. Simpson and K. Budd, (ed.) *Cancer Pain Management: A Comprehensive Approach* (Chapter 1). Maidenhead: Oxford University Press.

Simpson, K.H. (2000), Philosophy of cancer pain management, in K.H. Simpson and K. Budd, (ed.) *Cancer Pain Management: A Comprehensive Approach* (Chapter 1). Maidenhead: Oxford University Press.

Singla, S., Marwah, N. and Dutta, S. (2008) Congenital insensitivity to pain (hereditary sensory and autonomic neuropathy type V): a rare case report, *Journal of Dentistry for Children,* 75: 207–11.

Sutton, L.M., Porter, L.S. and Keefe, F.J. (2002) Cancer pain at the end of life: a biopsychosocial perspective, *Pain* 99: 5–10.

Wall, P. (1999) *Pain: The Science of Suffering* (pp. 29–30). London: Orion Publishing Group.

Welsh Health Planning Forum (1992) *Protocol for Investment in Health Gain: Pain, Discomfort and Palliative Care.* Cardiff: NHS Directorate.

White, A.K. (2000) Men making sense of their chest pain – niggles, doubts and denials, *Journal of Clinical Nursing,* 9(4): 534–41.

Williams, A.C. (2002) Facial expression of pain: an evolutionary account, *Behavioral and Brain Sciences,* 25(4): 439–55.

World Health Organization (1980) *International Classification of Impairments, Disabilities and Handicaps* Geneva: World Health Organization.

Dilemmas in pain management

2

Chapter contents

Introduction
Principles
Moral and ethical principles
Effects of illness on moral behaviour
Morals and pain
Deontology
Utilitarianism
Performing a moral calculus
   Quality adjusted life year (QALY) calculations
Rights and duties

Bioethics
   Autonomy
   Beneficence
   Nonmaleficence
   Justice
The best way to organize pain management
Considering the particular nature of pain in developing principles of managing pain
Summary
Reflective activity
References
Further reading

Introduction

In this chapter we examine some of the key underlying ethical principles of pain management. In order to do this we explore just what we mean by the idea of principles. How knowledge of ethics should influence our pain management practice and to what extent the care that organizations deliver is shaped by consideration of these principles. As part of this chapter we consider three case studies that will provide you with an opportunity to explore the fundamental principles in action.

There are nine broad areas covered in this chapter. They are:

1. principles and moral and ethical principles;
2. effects of illness on moral behaviour;
3. deontology;
4. utilitarianism;
5. rights and duties;
6. bioethics;
7. rights for people in pain;
8. organizing pain management;
9. developing principles of pain management.

As a result the following objectives will be addressed:

- Define the underlying values that should inform practice when caring for someone in pain.
- Evaluate the effect that adopting these values will have on practice.

Principles

If we are to explore the underlying values that should inform the practice of managing pain, then we need to examine the ethical principles on which these values are based. In order to do this we need to define what we mean when we talk about principles.

Activity 2.1

Think about the word 'principle' – what does it mean to you? Take time to write down a definition.

If we look up principle in a dictionary we get the following definitions:

> **1 a:** a comprehensive and fundamental law, doctrine, or assumption.
> **b**(1): a rule or code of conduct (2): habitual devotion to right principles 'a man of principle'.
> **c:** the laws or facts of nature underlying the working of an artificial device.
> **2:** a primary source: ORIGIN.
> **3 a:** an underlying faculty or endowment 'such principles of human nature as greed and curiosity'.
> **b:** an ingredient (as a chemical) that exhibits or imparts a characteristic quality.
> **In principle:** with respect to fundamentals.
> (Merriam Webster Online, 2008)

Principle therefore refers to three concepts.

- The first relates to underpinning rules or codes that dictate the best way to do something. In other words there is a moral or an ethical dimension to the best way to manage pain.
- The second relates to the organization of dealing with pain. There is a best way to organize care and

treatments and this is the most effective way to deal with pain.
- The third relates to the particular nature of pain and the most appropriate way of dealing with the restrictions imposed by this.

Moral and ethical principles

Morality is formed from the ideas about right and wrong conduct held by a society. Within any society there are likely to be a range of values and ideas about what is right and what is wrong among most members of that society; there will be a workable consensus of what is acceptable. This consensus or 'norm' forms the basis for daily dealing with other members of that society. To fail to uphold them is to live outside of the normal standard expected of a member of that society. Mild transgressions are frowned on as rudeness or a lack of consideration whereas major transgressions are viewed as criminal behaviour or sins, particularly in religious cultures, and attract retribution in some form or other. Learning about our own culture's moral norms is an important part of growing up (Beauchamp and Childress, 2008).

Effects of illness on moral behaviour

Illnesses can cause people to behave in an 'immoral fashion' unless allowances are made for the illness. Mental health problems are a good example of this; diseases such as schizophrenia, anorexia nervosa and alcoholism all pose the risk for the sufferer of unwittingly transgressing moral norms in both mild (e.g. talking to oneself) and major (e.g. self-harm) ways. Because of its overriding nature pain can also cause people to become morally vulnerable, more so if the pain is chronic, through failure to interact appropriately with others, the anger it can precipitate or the drive to seek remedies for the pain. We explore the nature of chronic pain in more depth in Chapter 8. Here we focus on an example of moral issues illustrated in the following case study.

Case study 2.1: Chronic pain medication: a moral dilemma?

Christine Walker is a 34-year-old lady with a loving supporting husband and three children. The youngest is 3 years old. For eight years she has suffered from chronic low back pain ever since an occupational injury, the consequences of which had left her with sufficient compensation to not have to work but dependent on large doses of opioid-based co-analgesics. The effect of this was to make her drowsy and anxious without really easing her pain. She continued to take them because they were all that was on offer from her general practitioner and if she took enough she was able to get some sleep. Since watching a TV programme on medical uses of cannabis she has started to experiment with smoking cannabis and has found that she now very rarely needs to take her prescribed analgesia. She is very careful that her children do not see her smoking the cannabis but feels that the legal risks are well worth it because she is a lot happier, has less pain, is now able to deal with a lot of problems at home she previously avoided. Her relationship with her children and husband has also improved. She has however been cautioned for possession of cannabis and is worried that she now has a criminal record.

In the case study above Christine has responded to her pain in a manner that puts her at risk morally because she has had to break the law to achieve some improvement in her condition. There are many people in pain who are faced with similar problems. Consider Christine's story:

1. What moral lessons can be drawn from it?
2. What would you do as a health professional if a patient/client asked you whether they should start taking cannabis?
3. What would you do if a patient/client you were caring for disclosed to you that they were actively using this drug?

Christine's case illustrates the link between moral and legal issues. She has found some relief from her pain and this is the most important ethical point. On the other hand 'the law is the law', and using cannabis does break the law and so the consequences for one person need to be weighed in the balance of the consequences for society as a whole (a utilitarian approach). You might also feel that to break the law, no matter how good the reason, is wrong and that you should not be seen to condone this position (a deontological approach).

Another position you might take would depend on your sense of professional ethics. These are encoded in various official and unofficial codes of conduct. There might even be conflict between various professional rules. For example, you might feel that as a health professional you have a responsibility to work within the law and that failure to do so is a serious breach of professional ethics.

The presence of children may be an important consideration. The impact of smoking cannabis could be viewed as a negative influence – exposure to criminal behaviour, or positive – improved parenting as a result of better symptom control.

These are all sound ethical viewpoints, they can be logically argued and defended and those taking one perspective may feel strongly that they are in the right whereas the other is in the wrong. Your beliefs will be shaped by a number of influencing factors.

As a health professional we have a duty to support our patients in any way that helps them ease their pain. You may feel so strongly that you advocate the legalization of cannabis regardless of the effect these actions might have on your professional status and credibility. Alternatively, you might feel that as a health professional you should discourage your patients/clients from breaking the law. You recognize that they are morally vulnerable and as a consequence may make decisions that they would regret if they were not in pain. This might be fuelled by concern that smoking cannabis can give rise to other health problems, such as respiratory and mental illnesses.

Another position you could take is that as a health

professional you must abide by the law as you have a wider responsibility to the general public and society as a whole and also to your profession.

Health carers may seek a compromise position, that is, as long as you see no harm coming to anyone you might support the decision 'off the record'. However, they have asked you for advice and this therefore begs the question 'can you ever be off the record as a health care professional?' Where the wishes and desires of others conflict with our own deeply held beliefs, then it is possible to take a position that respects the position of one party while maintaining one's own personal principles. This position is held by the conscientious objector. When adopting this stand you are in essence refusing to act yourself but are doing so in a way that does not impose conditions or obstructions on others to help. This is a perfectly legitimate and acceptable line to take as long as it does not transgress your normal professional role. This position requires recognition that the right of a person, in this case the client, to decide what is best for them should not override another person's right, the health professional's, to decide what is best for themselves.

The disclosure of illegal drug use raises some additional ethical concerns, the first of which is confidentiality. We have an obligation to respect patient confidentiality. Various legal cases have recognized the legitimacy of confidentiality between doctors and patients/client for example but within limitations. One of these is that the doctor should not knowingly withhold information that could lead to harm to others and therefore a judgement concerning likelihood of harm would be a consideration as to whether the right to confidentiality be broken. Another issue with respect to confidentiality is the need to consider who should have access to this confidential information and if and where this information is recorded. For example, are you going to make an entry in the patient's medical notes or are you going to inform the wider health care team whose members may have differing concerns to you, such as a social worker or in Christine's case the health visitor? Many pain clinics keep separate notes on patients that contain such confidential information, in much the same way that mental health notes are often kept separate from general medical notes.

An additional consideration is the effect of disclosure of information on the therapeutic relationship between you and your client/patient. A basis for confidentiality is that you have been trusted with this personal and important information and this could be threatened if you disclose this information. A way around this problem is to set ground rules for the disclosure of information. If you explain to the patient from the outset that information needs to be shared within the health care team, this can redress the balance as it gives the patient/client the opportunity to consider whether or not to continue.

Of course all of this discussion ignores a fundamental ethical issue with regard to Christine's case; that is, has she had the best care so far? Her only treatment seems to have been a long-term prescription of co-analgesics. You may feel that this is an inappropriate medical intervention and has contributed or even caused Christine's moral dilemma. In other words her problem is at least partly iatrogenic.

Morals and pain

The way people respond to pain is frequently used as a judgement on their ability to lead a proper moral life. For example, for centuries endurance of pain and suffering has been seen as a Christian ideal because Christ was crucified and suffered. The Judaeo-Christian faiths like many other forms of religious belief, such as mysticism, shamanism, Taoism and Hinduism, see pain as a means to gain closer spiritual identification with a God or the Gods. Pain serves as a punishment for sin, a cure for disease, a weapon against the body and its desires, or a means by which the ego may be transcended and spiritual sickness healed, a way to get closer to God.

> **Key point**
>
> A more complete overview of pain from a Christian perspective can be found by reading C.S. Lewis's book *The Problem of Pain*, Fount Paperbacks.

Religious philosophy balances these beliefs by advocating care of those suffering as a moral ideal. An example of this is traditional Judaism's prescriptive laws of *bikkur holim,* or visiting the sick (Nutkiewicz, 2002). This is of course a simplistic statement of a complex approach and we should acknowledge that many religions recognize shades of behaviour we are unable to consider here.

One of the moral problems we face and which religion offers an answer for is; 'who or what decides what is right or wrong?' Of course, this begs the question 'what is right or wrong?' There are several different ways of coming to an answer for this question.

The first is to take an *absolutist position*. This is a prevalent way of addressing moral issues, particularly in the Western world. A dominant example of such an approach is taken by many religious groups. Here the moral values of right or wrong might be translated into the values of *good* and *evil*. A right moral act is one that is good and a wrong moral act is evil. However, even with this position we run into a major problem that has troubled ethical philosophers for centuries. This can be encapsulated as follows:

Is an act good only if it results in an outcome that is good?

or

Does good only occur if the actions taken are in themselves good?

Activity 2.2

When you are dealing with others do you take the first position 'an act is good only if it results in an outcome that is good' a crude way of stating this might be 'the ends justify the means', or do you take the opposite position that 'good only occurs if the actions taken are in themselves good?'

Try to be honest and think about your dealings with your friends and family and not just your professional relationships. For example, if you have children do you ever shout at them? If you do would you tell them off for shouting at each other or at you?

You might be someone who adopts an absolutist stand and always follows the second position; you might therefore consider that the way you act is far more important than the results of your actions. If you do your position is shared by a school of ethical philosophy known as deontology.

If however you take the first position in your dealings with others, you will have followed the utilitarianist approach to ethics. You may well have found that your own practical ethics adopted a varied approach depending on the situation and context you found yourself in. This is often the case for many people.

Deontology

Deontology is essentially a rules-based system of ethics that has at its heart the values of *obligation* or *duty* and the *rightness* of acts. The word deontology is Greek for the 'science of duty'. At its heart is the idea that only by fulfilling your obligations to another through your actions towards them can you be ethically correct. These obligations or duties are shaped by universal independent principles, and hard line deontologists argue that only by sticking to them in your actions will you be ethical in your practice independent of their ends or consequences. Therefore, as long as you act correctly the consequences of your action on the individual or yourself have no relevance to the ethical morality of this position. This is a particularly useful philosophy to use when you cannot be sure of the outcome.

Key point

Deontology

Duty is the foundation of morality; an act is either morally right or wrong in itself irrespective of the consequences.

The universal independent principles are also known as categorical imperatives. The leading philosopher in this school of thought was Immanuel Kant and his ideas published in the eighteenth century can be summed up as:

- Man is essentially a rational being therefore emotions should be ruled out of moral actions.

- You should do what is right, because it is right and for no other reason.
- The outcome of an action is not decisive, but the motive behind the act is what counts; that is, having the right intention makes an action good.
- To act in a way you would be naturally inclined to, by upbringing for example, does not make your actions deserve credit even when they concur with what duty demands.
- You should act in a way that you would desire to be a universal law that governs everybody's actions.
- You should do your duty regardless of the consequences.
- If you take an action that will benefit you then it cannot be a moral action.
- Unthinking obedience to an external moral authority that conflicts with your personal moral conviction is not a moral position.
- There must always be a personal conviction that the action is right.

Kant's ideas suggest principles that would be applied in every situation. The sorts of principle that have been suggested include:

- Do others no harm.
- Do not lie.
- Respect others.
- Never break your promises.

Whatever principles a Kantian deontologist has they will be strongly held personal beliefs. They may differ between individuals or the interpretation or translation of these beliefs into actions may differ because of factors such as culture and upbringing. Even two apparently similar principles may conflict with each other if care is not taken. For example, the principle 'always tell the truth' and 'do not lie' may seem to be the same but in practice holding to the first may mean that you feel you have a responsibility to volunteer the truth without prompting while the latter would mean that you tell the truth when asked but would not necessarily volunteer it. This can have many implications in everyday life as well as clinical practice.

Deontological principles will always be tested when put into context. For example, you are caring for a patient who has just been diagnosed with a terminal disease and is experiencing severe pain. The relatives are insistent that the patient should not be informed of their terminal disease. You and the members of the health care team have to decide whether or not to accede to these demands and lie to the patient about the cause of their pain so that the patient will remain ignorant of their illness.

If you held the principle 'do not lie' to be a universal law what would you do?

According to the Kantian approach to deontology, it would be entirely permissible to accede to these wishes if you were to accept the premise that lying should be universally acceptable in all situations. If you cannot accept this then lying would not be justified. But is there ever a situation where lying is acceptable? Sometimes there may be situations where there is conflict between moral principles, for example, *do not lie* and *do not harm*. You may consider that by telling the patient the truth you will by the same action inflict harm.

If you do this you are ascribing a hierarchy to your principles. In other words, you are saying that some principles are more universal than others.

Key points

Kant's theory

STRENGTHS

- Universal maxims are clear
- Humanistic approach
- Respect for others
- Universal application limits self-interest

WEAKNESSES

- Conflicts of duty can often arise
- Does not readily allow exceptions to be made

According to Kant there are no prescribed 'moral' actions, only ways of defining moral actions. Furthermore, for Kant, the decisive factor in whether or not an action was moral is the personal conviction of the one who had to take the action. Thus, it is entirely possible that people could conscientiously arrive at totally opposite choices of action in the same situation, depending on all sorts of outside factors, like upbringing, personal experience, culture, and so on.

The underlying concepts supporting Kant's ethic are.

- *Respect for persons*: Kantian ethics advocate respect for the person through ensuring we always treat them as ends and not as means.
- *Equality*: universal laws mean that we must apply the same principle in every situation thus everybody, including ourselves and our loved ones, are treated in the same way.
- *Liberty*: you have to be free to think for yourself in order to arrive at your universal laws
- *Rationality*: You must have reasoned out your universal laws and not be acting out of an emotional or experiential response to events.

Deontology has been criticized as being formalized and inflexible as it relies on rigid rules and fails to consider differences between cases or be responsive to the context. It has also been seen as too abstract to guide action in the field.

Other models of deontology (absolutism and natural law) exist where rules of behaviour are prescribed for others to follow. These run the risk of removing individual responsibility because they are based on notions of duty imposed from outside and not self-imposed by the individual and are often tied up with punishments or forms of coercion to ensure compliance.

Utilitarianism

Utilitarianism is an influential view of ethics that comes from the teleological or consequentialist school of ethics. It was first formulated by Jeremy Bentham in the early nineteenth century and developed later by John Stuart Mill later in that century. It opposes many of the key principles of deontological ethics because at its heart is the concept that the value of the action lies not in the act itself, but in its result. According to utilitarianism what is important is the result or outcome and not how it is achieved.

Key concepts in utilitarianism are:

- pleasure;
- happiness;
- freedom;
- doing good;
- knowledge;
- beauty;
- justice.

Key point

Utilitarianism

A school of ethics that holds that actions can be judged to be right or wrong based on their outcomes and the amount of happiness that is generated for all those concerned.

In general terms utilitarianism can be summarized as actions are considered *intrinsically good* if they produce maximum pleasure for the majority of people affected. A commonly heard way of expressing this concept is the idea of 'the greatest happiness to the greatest number'.

Performing a moral calculus

Utilitarianism requires you to calculate the following for each course of action:

- Identify everyone who would be affected by the action and its consequences.
- Determine whether they benefit from the action or are disadvantaged by the action.
- Determine the extent to which they are advantaged or disadvantaged.
- Sum up all the positives and negatives.
- Choose the option that produces the maximum amount of common good.

Utilitarianism invites the use of individual reason and judgement, giving some autonomy in choice of actions. However, you have to apply utilitarianism carefully in practice as it is not simply a matter of maximizing pleasure and benefit for those on whom the actions will bear but of weighing up the consequences of doing this as well. An example that helps to explain this follows.

Case study 2.2: Sarah Sobers

There is only a finite amount of money available for spending on health care. In the UK most of this money is raised through taxation to fund the NHS. This imposes restrictions on how much can be spent on various treatments. Consider the following case of Mrs Sarah Sobers, a 50-year-old, who has been diagnosed with advanced breast cancer. She has had a mastectomy and three courses of standard chemotherapy which have not succeeded in reducing the spread of the metastatic disease. This is causing her moderate bone pain.

A new experimental oncology drug treatment has just been made available and Sarah matches the profile for its use. The drug costs £15,000 for each treatment and Sarah will require monthly treatments for six months at a total cost of £90,000. It is anticipated that this treatment, although having unpleasant side-effects, should reduce Sarah's pain experience and improve her quality of life, although only extending it by two years. The alternative is to be referred to palliative care services where her pain will be effectively managed and she will be assured of a peaceful death. In this case her prognosis would be that she would die within six months.

Sarah is married to David and they have no children although their nephew Barry, aged 15, lives with them. She is a popular member of her community and is an inspirational and well-loved secondary school teacher. Sarah cannot afford to pay for this treatment privately.

For the same cost, six people of the same age could have a total hip replacement which would reduce the moderate degree of pain they have as a result of chronic arthritis and restore their mobility. This would greatly improve their quality of life. The prognosis from a hip replacement is up to 20 years of good function and no hip pain. The alternative is they spend these years in increasing pain and immobility.

Consider the above case study and perform a moral calculus to determine the choice an utilitarian approach to ethics might make. In so doing consider the following questions:

- Identify everyone who would be affected by the action and its consequences.
- Determine whether they benefit from the action or are disadvantaged by the action.
- Determine the extent to which they are advantaged or disadvantaged.
- Sum up all the positives and negatives.
- Choose the option that produces the maximum amount of common good.

This is a moral dilemma that many health care professionals and health services face when determining how to allocate resources and while our example is oversimplified, it does allow an exploration of utilitarianist approaches to health costs. Admittedly, it is very crude but we have performed our moral calculus.

Sarah is obviously affected by this decision but who else would be? We can include her family but also the clinicians who are caring for Sarah. In addition, we can consider the impact on her local community and the children she has taught over the years. There is also an impact on society as a whole. Do we want to be considered members of a society that would allow someone to die because of economic concerns?

Opposed to this we must consider the other group who are affected. Like Sarah, they have a debilitating condition, one which causes them an equivalent degree of pain but will not kill them although their lack of mobility significantly affects their well-being. These six people will also have families and people who love them. We have not given their personal details but we can assume that some of them will be currently working and might have several people depending on them as a result of their work. If they were to give up work because of their disability this would have knock-on effects that are not just personal but impact on wider society. In economic terms alone they would be going from a net contributor to society to a dependant as they no longer paid taxes but received benefits instead.

Sarah would clearly benefit from the treatment, her life would be extended by 18 months at least and also her quality of life would improve as her pain reduces although this must be outweighed by the side-effects of the new drug treatment. It is hard to quantify these outcomes in terms of benefits and disadvantages as we are dealing with a person's life. If Sarah does not have the treatment she will die sooner but her death will be pain free and peaceful. We have the advantage of years of clinical experience and effective palliative care to ensure that she does not suffer needlessly. However, whatever the immediate gain in two years time Sarah is likely to die despite having the expensive drug treatment and she will eventually need this good palliative care, so it can perhaps be discounted from our calculation. Sarah's husband and nephew benefit because their much loved wife and aunt is alive for much longer. There would be a benefit for society as someone who has committed themselves to bettering society through her actions as a teacher is helped to live for a longer period of time.

However, the six people who have a hip replacement will also benefit and their benefit will last for much longer. Weighed up against this is the inconvenience and pain of having their hip surgery and the risks that are associated with this. This will have consequences for their families and society and not just in terms of financial benefits.

Some of these benefits are huge and therefore offer great advantage; for example, the prolonged life span for Sarah and the improved quality of life benefits for both groups. Others are small or of less value and some are so ethereal that they are difficult to assign value to; the impact on the children Sarah taught for example. However, the moral dilemma underpinning these two choices is what is the cost of one life? It is difficult to make these calculations. How do you weigh up the gains of the two sides?

One group will have 120 years of pain relief as opposed to two years, a 60-fold improvement in pain and quality of life. There will therefore be significantly more pain relief as a result. Opposed to this is the fact that Sarah will live for longer, her prognosis is four times longer if she has the drug treatment,

whereas we are unable to say that the life span of the other group will improve.

Quality adjusted life year (QALY) calculations

There are economic formulae that are designed to do just this. One example is the QALY, which is used by the National Institute for Health and Clinical Excellence (NICE) in the UK to make judgements on the best effective treatments for a condition. It forms the basis of real clinical decision-making rather than this example. A QALY is a form of moral calculus. It asks the questions:

> How many years extra life will the treatment provide this patient?
> What will the quality of those extra years be?
> How expensive is this treatment?
> (Herring, 2006: 531)

Herring (2006) reports that where a treatment cost exceeds £35,000 then NICE must also consider additional reasons such as wider societal costs and benefits and the innovative nature of the technology.

On this basis it could be argued that if the experimental drug treatment represents a breakthrough in technology, then it might be justified to support its use on the grounds that future patients might receive cheaper and more effective care.

Based on this calculus what is the correct thing to do? We would probably err on the side of the six hip replacements but we feel very uncomfortable doing this and would be happy to follow NICE guidelines on the use of the new drug.

In summary, utilitarianism asks you to examine the common good and not just the good to the individuals or potential individuals concerned. The impact on the whole of society has to be considered. This has wider, negative impacts for society than the immediate benefits for a small group of people. Consider the following questions.

(1) Do you wish to live in a society that uses these sorts of moral argument to make distinctions between life and death and suffering?

(2) What does this case study tell us about respect for others and individual rights?

(3) Can we make a distinction between individual benefit as opposed to benefits to the greater good?

(4) Would we feel differently if we were discussing a non-health-related issue, such as the rights of an individual to express their beliefs and the offence these beliefs might cause to a large section of our society?

There are different forms of utilitarianism (comprehensive or act utilitarianism and organizational or rule-based utilitarianism) which view this school of ethics from different perspectives. Our *Further reading* section at the end of this chapter will guide you to suitable texts.

> **Key point**
>
> *Utilitarianism*
>
> STRENGTHS
>
> - Straightforward
> - Common sense
> - Can be quantified and measured
>
> WEAKNESSES
>
> - Difficult and unwieldy to apply
> - Rules conflict or decisions differ in different situations
> - Who decides what is good?
> - Who should be included in the moral calculus?
> - Who does the calculations?
> - It can reduce people to numbers and financial units.

Rights and duties

The two main ethical approaches described above have introduced you to several core ideas that should help you identify some principles for helping people in pain. These can be thought of in terms of rights and duties.

The basic rights that these two schools of ethical philosophy would award patients/clients and their families and your duty towards them revolve around the following themes:

- *Doing the 'right thing' for those in need*: how you do this may differ of course. You may wish to focus on producing a good outcome for them or on making sure that whatever the outcomes your actions are good.
- *Respect for the person*: this may involve recognition of the freedom of the individual to do what is right for them or it may manifest as recognizing that it is a person you are dealing with and not a symptom or a number or a monetary unit.
- *Helping and minimizing harm*: the concept of doing good is different to the concept of doing the right thing. It is about ensuring happiness and pleasure and avoiding situations that would cause harm. It requires a judgement on what is best for the patients well-being.
- *Justice and equality*: the concept of justice is key to ensuring that people are treated fairly and that each individual would expect the same standard of care and treatment.

Bioethics

In the field of ethics related to health care bioethics, a set of guiding principles have been developed in response to addressing the particular thorny issue of who should decide health care problems, the patient/client or the health professional. In adults who are mentally competent and conscious this would seem to be a straightforward case of the patient deciding. However, as we know, many people who are ill rely on the knowledge, judgement, skills, experiences and decisions of a wide range of health professionals; this puts them at the mercy of the actions of their carers. There are four bioethical principles that have been put forward as a way to act that prevents abuse of this power (Beauchamp and Childress, 2008), which are as follows:

- autonomy;
- beneficence;
- nonmaleficence;
- justice.

Autonomy

Autonomy is about respect for the decision-making capacity of an autonomous person. An autonomous individual is someone who has *capacities of self governance, such as understanding, reasoning,*

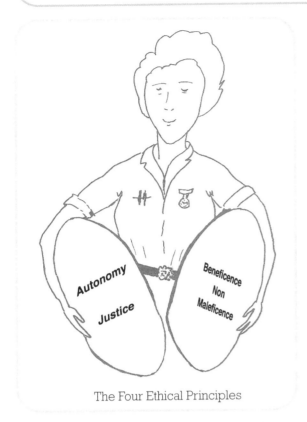

The Four Ethical Principles

examples given this may be done by statutory laws or judicial review. However, it may also occur in more normal situations; for example, where someone is deemed to be a person of diminished autonomy (cognitively challenged individuals).

Impact of pain on autonomy

In an earlier discussion we looked at the impact pain can have in making an individual morally vulnerable. We need to consider whether it has the same impact on the ability of someone in pain to make an autonomous decision. It could be argued that the person in pain has lost or diminished their autonomy because it drives them to take actions they might otherwise not have taken, such as desiring health professionals to remove their pain by whatever means available even if it is not the most appropriate choice for them. As Lisson (1987: 649–59) suggests:

> *Pain is dehumanizing. The severer the pain, the more it overshadows the patient's intelligence . . . Pain destroys autonomy: the patient is afraid to make the slightest movement. All choices are focused on either relieving the present pain or preventing greater future pain . . .*

deliberating, managing and independent choosing (Beauchamp and Childress, 2008: 100). In other words, autonomy is about respecting an individual's independence and recognizing their competence in making decisions for themselves.

As we have seen in our earlier discussion of conscientious objection, respect for autonomy in decision-making gives priority to the values and wishes of the individual as long as they do not adversely affect the rights of others.

In health care, the issue of informed consent lies at the heart of any discussion of autonomy. The patient or client who is capable of making a conscious, deliberate decision on a proposed treatment after being apprised of its risks and benefits has the right to grant or deny permission for it to go ahead. The intention of informed consent and respect for autonomy is to make the patient or client both a partner in decision-making and a consumer (Farber Post et al., 1996).

When an individual's wishes are obscure, inaccessible, or subject to competing principles, between two parties for example, as in the case of separation of conjoined twins or termination of pregnancy, that judgement of others may be substituted. In the

If a person is in severe pain we can suppose that they are incapacitated in their ability to make decisions and are also probably incapacitated in their freedom to make decisions. However, this gives rise to the question of whether incapacity means that there is no need to offer a choice. When we respect the autonomy of a capable individual we are empowering them and honouring their right to self-determination. In a person with diminished capability, failure to act to relieve the pain is a failure to remove the cause of their incapability. It prevents us from empowering the individual and encouraging them to make decisions for themselves. In this way allowing someone who has no capability to make a choice to be in pain when you have the means to prevent this is a form of neglect as well as indicating a lack of compassion and humanness (Farber Post et al., 1996).

The default value for pain management in people with diminished capacity for autonomy ought therefore to be to treat the pain. However, there is a large body of evidence that heath carers fail to adequately manage pain in children (Nagy, 1998) and the elderly and mentally ill (Hayes 1995; Rakel and Herr, 2004). This does not mean that people working in these fields of health care do not hold the moral belief that the humane response is to relieve pain but it is to recognize that often even experienced health workers:

- are unable to assess the signs of pain (including verbal and non-verbal signs) (Carr and Mann, 2008);
- judgments about pain are as influenced by socio-cultural factors, including age, gender, race, and ethnicity (Farber Post et al., 1996);
- are also influenced by professional culture to take decisions for vulnerable people.

Another reason for providing pain relief when someone who is in pain is incapable of making a decision is that pain relief in the form of *'analgesia is routinely given when patients are understood to be in pain'* (Farber Post et al., 1996; 354). In other words, pain relief is the normal treatment for people in pain. This makes the omission of pain relief not only inhumane but irrational as well.

Competent refusal of pain relief

However, there are times when competent people may refuse analgesia. They may do this for a number of reasons. Some may choose not to have high doses of a drug or be changed to more potent analgesia for example. They may do so because:

- they are worried about obscuring their *'intellectual and emotional awareness'* (Farber Post et al., 1996);
- they may be concerned about avoiding the side-effects of the drug such as nausea or constipation;
- they may have fears about addiction;
- they may not trust health professionals;
- they may wish to prove to themselves their psychological or spiritual hardiness.

Whether or not we as health professionals agree with these motives is largely beside the point if we are to honour their autonomy because the choice they have made is a deliberate one. As the concept of autonomy focuses on self-determination and liberty as long as this does not interfere with the rights of others, it follows that if an individual prefers to experience pain and this harms no one else then they should be allowed to make this choice. However, we may wish to ensure that they are fully cognizant of the facts in order to make their choice. If someone has made a decision based on misconceptions then we should act to inform them of this even if they then decide to ignore this new information.

Limited autonomy

The concept of limited autonomy may be applied absolutely to someone with a learning disability for example, or on the basis of a sliding scale. Childhood is an excellent example of this. Autonomy in children is based on the concept of sufficient maturity of understanding. As a child grows they move through various phases of autonomy, until they reach adulthood. In practice each successive stage recognizes more liberty (freedom to act independently) and agency (capacity for intentional action) and is therefore less restrictive in practice although the growing person's awareness and perception of these differences may not recognize this and this may cause conflict between the individual and those in authority such as parents or teachers. This is an everyday example of dilemmas in autonomy.

Beneficence

Beneficence means doing good to others. It is the underlying reason why many health professionals become involved in the field of health care. They want to help others who are vulnerable in some way. It is particularly important where someone is incapable of making an autonomous decision or has a limited capability to do so.

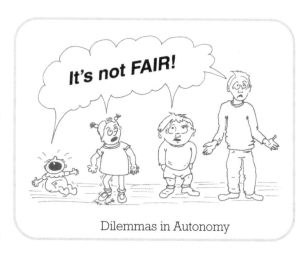

Dilemmas in Autonomy

A beneficence-centred approach to pain would apply where someone is unable to make a decision for themselves. The principle of beneficence informs us how to act when someone's wishes are unknown and/or they are unable to make a decision for themselves, perhaps because of severe illness or cognitive impairment. In this case a surrogate decision is made. This surrogate decision should be guided by the person's well-being. However, it should not be based on firm rules but individualized according to what is known about the person's beliefs and desires. This implicitly requires the involvement of those who know the person although it does not necessarily mean that what those people – family, friends, relatives and carers – want is necessarily the best thing for the person. If no agreement is obtained between the various interested parties then there is a need to seek help and advice and this is usually where a judicial decision on care might be sought.

Occasionally, it is impossible to know in advance someone's desires, perhaps because of the emergency nature of the situation. In such instances the tendency is to make a decision that opts for treatment because an assumption is made that most people would ordinarily want to receive treatment that would restore health or ease suffering. Faber Post et al. (1996) describe this as a default posture that supports treatment.

Nonmaleficence

Nonmaleficence refers to avoiding harm or doing no harm. This principle forces health professionals to consider the consequences of any actions and also to weigh up the results of doing nothing with the consequences of treatment. At times this can be a very straightforward easy decision. Someone admitted to hospital with a clear case of a ruptured appendix needs to be operated on as soon as possible, and this is reflected in the information given to the client or patient. The risks of a general anaesthetic and the discomfort after the surgery are more than outweighed by the benefits of emergency surgery. In other instances the issue may be less clear cut. For example, a man with widespread peripheral vascular disease who has a gangrenous leg may be a good candidate for an above-knee amputation. Poor general health status may mean that he could die from the effects of the

anaesthetic or the stress of surgery, and if he survives may have long-term health problems as a consequence of immobility that will shorten his life considerably. In this latter instance decisions are harder to make and depend on close collaboration between the patient/client their families and the health care team.

Justice

Justice refers to the principle of fairly distributing the risk, burdens and benefits of decision-making. This can be especially difficult where the intentions of the patient or client infringe on the autonomy of others. In such cases a judgement has to be made as to the most equitable outcome, the one that is fairest to the patient or client but also produces the least harm to others. This might seem straightforward but it is important to remember that justice has been interpreted in several different ways; for example, equal access to health care may mean that people with a greater need are discriminated against. Other viewpoints are that justice in health care should be given according to merit or contribution to society or effort to help oneself stay healthy or ability to pay. The ideal of justice has shaped the development of health organizations. Many European countries rely on a system of health care delivery based on equity; that is, treatment based on need and not on other aspects of merit, which could be argued as being discriminatory for example.

> ### Key point
>
> *Equality and equity*
>
> **Equality** refers to a situation where two or more different parties are treated as exactly the same, they are regarded as having the same worth and value and requiring the same rights.
> **Equity** refers to fairness. Two people may not be the same and therefore allowances need to be made to correct the differences between them.

Ethical considerations are often complex and as they reflect cultural beliefs they may vary widely.

When considering ethical principles we have to remember that while some may seem to take precedence over others this is not always the case and real life situations are usually far more complex. When applying ethics to pain many commentators tend to concentrate on life and death situations particularly in the terminally ill. While these are of course very important dilemmas with strong messages for all health workers, it is important to realize that ethical issues occur in pain management in a variety of settings.

One solution to this possible dilemma from the health professional's point of view is the *doctrine of double effect*. According to the doctrine of double effect if an intended good outcome also produces a bad side-effect this is ethically acceptable as long as this side-effect was not intended (Beauchamp and Childress, 2008: 162). This applies whether or not the side-effect is foreseeable or even likely to occur. This doctrine is used to justify the administration of high doses of opioids for the purpose of relieving suffering in the terminally ill. In Peter's case (see Case Study 2.3) he was given intravenous diamorphine in order to relieve his severe pain and also to help calm him down. In order to ascertain whether the doctrine of double effect has been met we have to be convinced that the following conditions apply:

- *The good outcome must be achieved independently of the bad one*: the reason for giving the intravenous diamorphine was to treat Peter's pain and allow his emergency care to proceed and the distress that this subsequently caused Peter was certainly not intended.
- *The undesired outcome must not be the means of achieving the good outcome*: this is the case; it was certainly not the intention to control Peter's pain through turning him back into a heroin addict.
- *The action must be appropriate*: Peter has very severe injuries and the administration of intravenous diamorphine is an appropriate intervention, certainly alternative options are limited; an epidural is doubtful because of the need to change his position and Peter's blood loss, a femoral nerve block would not ease the pelvic injuries and as he had difficulties communicating, Entonox would have been impossible to administer. A possible alternative would have been to give a different analgesic but this would still have been an opioid.
- *The action must be proportional to the cause*: once again the use of the intravenous route rather than any other route is indicated by the nature of the injuries and the need for rapid treatment.

There are however problems with using the *doctrine of double effect* as an argument to support the health professionals' decisions. It can be argued that we are responsible for all the consequences of our actions, whether they are anticipated or not. As a result we should take the moral responsibility for both the desired and undesired effect. Critics of the doctrine say that it is used as an excuse to deny the responsibility for unintended actions.

Of course, at the time of treatment the medical team in accident and emergency had no idea of Peter's past history; they were responding to his immediate needs and they had made the surrogate decision to treat him by administering intravenous diamorphine. Although a default position dictated by the duties of beneficence and nonmaleficence was taken, it would be very difficult to argue that this was the wrong position to take at that time.

We have therefore established that the medical team acted morally and also made the right decision. However, what about Peter's subsequent distress; is he justified in his position? Or by acting morally correctly at each stage, is the health care team absolved from worry about this.

Clearly, Peter's autonomy was violated; he was not asked for his consent despite requiring medical intervention. The grounds for this violation are sound; he was temporarily of diminished autonomy because of his injuries and his pain. To have left him would have been an unacceptable act of doing harm as he was losing blood and his condition could have deteriorated.

Peter might well have agreed to the treatment if he had been given enough information to make an informed decision despite his obvious aversion to having intravenous diamorphine. His distress occurs because of his fear that the administration of intravenous diamorphine will turn him back into an addict. The ongoing moral duty of the health care team

Case study 2.3: Peter's consent

Peter John aged 38 is brought into the accident and emergency department. He has been knocked off his bicycle on the way to work and has a crushed pelvis and injuries to both legs. He has lost a lot of blood and is in very severe pain and it is difficult to communicate with him or treat his injuries because of this. As his pain is obviously causing a great deal of distress and there is a need to calm him down so that urgent attention to his injuries can be given a surrogate decision is made to administer diamorphine intravenously.

Although Peter's pain is now well controlled his distress seems to have increased and he becomes abusive; he says that he has been doped against his will and threatens to sue the doctors, nurses and the hospital. His mother arrives and when he sees her he starts to cry and tells her it is not his fault and not to let them take his daughter away. The doctors and nurses in the accident and emergency department are bemused by this.

Peter's mother explains that until six months ago he was an intravenous drug abuser and his drug of choice was heroin (diamorphine). His ex-wife was also an addict and has had a stroke following an overdose. She is being cared for by her parents who are trying to gain custody of his 14-year-old daughter, Amy. He had a very traumatic time 'kicking his habit' and has only recently started to feel better. He is scared that giving him diamorphine will turn him back into an addict.

Activity 2.3

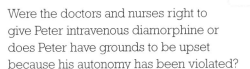

Were the doctors and nurses right to give Peter intravenous diamorphine or does Peter have grounds to be upset because his autonomy has been violated?

should be to ensure that he has the correct information about the use of diamorphine for pain relief and an appropriate pain management strategy to deal with his continuing care. Hopefully, this will reassure Peter and ease his distress. Of course, Peter will be a partner in the decision-making process from this point on because the pain relief has restored his capacity to make autonomous decisions. If the autonomous decision that is made is to refuse intravenous opioids in future this would have to be respected by the health care team and alternatives explored even though they may consider it to be the only reasonable option, which could be argued as being discriminatory.

Peter's case study illustrates the complexity of pain management and the potential conflicts that can occur. It also illustrates the challenges to offering ethically sound care. Health care professionals support the principles of autonomy, beneficence, nonmaleficence and justice although there is evidence within the literature that practice does not always conform to these principles. For example, there is a plethora of information that nurses and doctors underestimate and underassess the reports of acute pain from patients after surgery (Carr and Mann, 2008). This surely infringes a patient's autonomy. Many professionals continue to practise clinical interventions that are known to be ineffective while not introducing others they know to be effective (Walshe, 1998), therefore potentially doing harm.

The best way to organize pain management

Consideration of moral and ethical principles can be useful when it comes to deciding about the best way to organize pain management. During the 1990s authors such as Davey and Popay (1993) and Phillips et al. (1994) suggested that health care could be evaluated by considering criteria such as effectiveness, equity and efficiency with Davey and Popay (1993) recognizing the importance of the personal needs of individuals (humanity). These are criteria which form a useful basis for considering the delivery of health care in general and are important indicators in

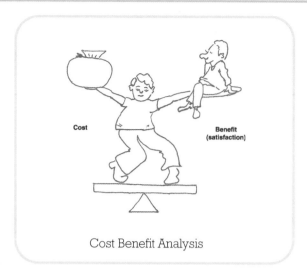

Cost Benefit Analysis

present-day governance (Sale, 2005) and health economics (Phillips, 2005); although authors such as Williams (2001) and Gwatkin et al. (2004) offer interesting examples of the complexity of health care provision and the dilemmas that can result in trying to ensure effective, humane, equitable and efficient health care.

Considering the particular nature of pain in developing principles of managing pain

When applying the above principles to pain we need to remember that pain is not a single entity but a complex condition that requires careful consideration before a plan of action is implemented. Failure to consider the true nature of pain that a person experi-

ences can cause false assumptions to be made; as we saw in the case of Christine, the possibly false assumption that co-analgesics alone can help her pain may have led to problems in her family and social life as well as turning to illegal activities. Assumptions such as this are commonly faced by people in pain. Interventions that are applicable to acute pains are often applied to chronic pain because people are unaware of alternatives or they are not readily available. Similarly, a lack of understanding of the physiology of pain might lead to a prescription of an opioid for an opioid resistance pain.

A true application of the principles would start by recognizing that:

- effectiveness depends on a deep understanding of the nature of pain;
- humanity requires an understanding of the interpersonal dimension of pain and the recognition of its unique effect on an individual;
- equity, that each person in pain has specific needs. Adopting a blanket approach to the problem of pain might not be the best thing to do and therefore a careful assessment of what those needs are is required;
- efficiency requires us to understand that the best approach for dealing with pain is not necessarily the cheapest, such as a prescription of paracetamol, or the most expensive, such as a highly technical procedure like radiofrequency lesion, although these might well be appropriate.

These principles need to be considered when planning and delivering ethical and appropriate care. This will be considered in later chapters.

Summary

In this chapter you have explored the foundations for determining the best way to care for people in pain. You have examined moral and ethical principles of pain management and have then looked at an overview of the guiding principles that organizations need to consider when delivering health care. This involved an introduction to some of the factors that need to be considered when addressing problems faced by people in pain. In this way you have explored the underlying values that should inform your practice and the practice of those around you when caring for someone in pain and have considered how these values should shape the care of the person in pain. These themes will be picked up and developed in the following chapters.

The main ideas we wished to communicate in this chapter were:

- Morality is formed from ideas about right and wrong.
- Illness, the pain experience, can impact on moral behaviour.

- Ideas of what constitute moral behaviour need to be examined from the perspective of a carer and the receiver of care.
- What constitutes ethical behaviour has been explored from different perspectives; the two leading schools being deontology and utilitarianism.
- Deontologists consider an act to be either morally right or wrong in itself irrespective of its consequence.
- Utilitarianism considers actions to be right or wrong based on their outcomes.
- There are strengths and limitations to both of these schools of thought.
- Nevertheless, they highlight basic rights and duties: doing the right thing for those in need; respect for the person; helping to minimize harm; justice and equality.
- Rights and duties are apparent within the four guiding principles of bioethics: autonomy; beneficence; nonmaleficence; and justice.
- The pain experience challenges the carer in the application of these principles.
- The best way to organize pain management services is to consider its effectiveness, equity, efficiency and how its delivery preserves humanity.

Reflective activity

As a conclusion to this chapter consider how knowledge of this theory will help you in your future practice. Try to be specific and use the following points/questions as a guide.

- *State* which elements of the chapter will help you in your future practice.
- *Elaborate:* be specific in terms of how this knowledge and understanding can be used in practice.
- *Give examples:* of care events which would benefit from what you have learnt.
- What are the *implications* if you change the way you practise.

You may prefer to use a reflective model such as Gibbs's (1988) to guide your reflection (see Appendix at the end of this book). Think of a specific example from your experiences as the starting point.

Describe the event and then proceed through the cycle. When analysing the situation draw on this chapter's theory to support your discussion and demonstrate your understanding.

References

Beauchamp, T.L. and Childress, J.F. (2008) *Principles of Biomedical Ethics*, 5th edn. Maidenhead: Oxford University Press.

Carr, E. and Mann, E. (2008) *Pain: Creative Approaches to Effective Management*, 2nd edn. London: Palgrave Macmillan.

Davey, B. and Popay, J. (1993) *Dilemmas in Health Care*, revised edn. Health Disease Series, (Chapter 1). Maidenhead: Open University Press.

Farber Post, L., Blustein, J., Gordon, E. and Neveloff Duber, N. (1996) Pain: ethics, culture, and informed consent to relief, (1996) *Journal of Law, Medicine & Ethics*, 24(4): 348–59. Available online at www.aslme.org/research/mayday/24.4/24.4h.php (accessed 22 June 2009).

Gibbs, G. (1988) *Learning by Doing: A Guide to Teaching and Learning Methods*. Oxford: Further Education Unit, Oxford Polytechnic.

Gwatkin, D.R., Bhuiya, A. and Victora, C.G. (2004) Making health systems more equitable, *The Lancet*, 364(9441): 1273–80.

Hayes, R. (1995) Pain assessment in the elderly, *British Journal of Nursing*, 4(20): 1199–204.

Herring, J. (2006) *Medical Law and Ethics* (Chapter 10). Oxford: Oxford University Press.

Hicks, C. (1998) The randomised control trial: a critique, *Nurse Researcher*, 6: 19–32.

Lisson, E.L. (1987) Ethical issues related to pain control, *Nursing Clinics North America*, 22(3): 649–59.

Merriam Webster Online (2008) www.merriam-webster.com/dictionary/principle (accessed 7 July 2008).

Nagy, S. (1998) Comparison of the effects on patients' pain on nursing working in burns and neonatal intensive care units, *Journal of Advanced Nursing*, 27(2): 335–40.

Nutkiewicz, M. (2002) Towards an ethic of suffering: a rejoinder to Jamie Mayerfeld, *American Pain Society Bulletin*, 12(6). Available online at www.ampainsoc.org/pub/bulletin/nov02/path1.htm (accessed 22 June 2009).

Phillips C. (2005) *Health Economics: An Introduction for Health Professionals*. Oxford: Blackwell Publishing.

Phillips, C., Palfrey, C., and Thomas, P. (1994) *Evaluating Health and Social Care*. Basingstoke: Macmillan Press.

Pope John Paul II (1984) *Salvifici Doloris*. Apostolic Letter Salvifici Doloris of the Supreme Pontiff John Paul II to the Bishops, to the Priests, to the Religious Families and to the Faithful of the Catholic Church on the Christian meaning of Human Suffering, Catholic Truth Society.

Rakel, B. and Herr, K. (2004) Assessment and treatment of postoperative pain in older adults, *Journal of PeriAnesthesia Nursing*, 19(3): 194–208.

Sale, D. (2005) *Understanding Clinical Governance and Quality Assurance*. Basingstoke: Palgrave Macmillan.

Walshe, K. (1998) Evidence based practice: a new area in health care? in P. Spurgeon (ed.) *The New Face of the NHS*, 2nd edn. London: Royal Society of Medicine.

Williams, A. (2001) Dilemmas in health care: responding to economic constraints in C. Komaromy (ed.) *Dilemmas in UK Health Care* (pp. 21–40), Maidenhead: Open University Press.

Further reading

American Pain Foundation (2009) *Pain Care Bill of Rights*. Available online: at *www.painfoundation.org/Publications/BORenglish.pdf* (accessed 18 June 2009).

Clinical Standards Advisory Group (1994) *Back Pain*. London: HMSO.

Lewis, C.S. (1940) *The Problem of Pain*. Fount Paperbacks.

Pope John Paul II (1984) *Salvifici Doloris*. Apostolic Letter Salvifici Doloris of the Supreme Pontiff John Paul II to the Bishops, to the Priests, to the Religious Families and to the Faithful of the Catholic Church on the Christian meaning of Human Suffering, Catholic Truth Society.

Communicating the experience of pain

3

Chapter contents

Introduction
Intrapersonal perspective of pain
Biopsychosocial model and communication
The intrapersonal nature of pain
   Nociceptive pain
   Gate control theory of pain
   Nociceptive transmission
Detection and modulation
Cutaneous receptors
Visceral receptors
Inflammation and primary hyperalgesia
Action potentials
Sensory nerve communication
The pain gate
   Descending mechanisms
   Neurotransmitters
   Secondary hyperalgesia
Ascending pathway
The brain
   Reticular formation
   Thalamus
   Cortex

Differing pain experiences
   Neuropathic pain
   Sensitization
   Abnormal impulses
   Amplification
   Sympathetically maintained pains
     (SMPs)
   Abnormal central processing
   Central pain
   Mixed nociceptive/neuropathic pain
   Complex pain sensation
Interpersonal pain
Influences on pain responses
   A sociocommunication model of pain
The pain experience
   Expression of pain
   Assessment or attribution of pain
   Actions
   The language of pain
Something lost in the translation
Iatrogenic communication
Summary
Reflective activity
References

Introduction

The focus of this chapter is communicating the pain experience. This we will consider in two broad ways. First, communicating the pain experience within the individual. This section of the chapter concentrates on the physiological and pathophysiological mechanisms involved in the sensation we call 'pain'. And second, communicating with people who are experiencing pain. This section of the chapter focuses on the external communication process.

It is not our intention to offer a comprehensive discussion of either the normal and abnormal physiology, or general communication theory. Both of these topics are covered well in many other resources which we reference at the end of this chapter.

The intent here is to offer an overview of the physiological and communication processes and to focus on aspects more specifically related to the pain experience. As a result we are making some assumptions here; that is, you have some understanding of nervous system physiology and communication theory.

There are three broad areas that will be covered in this chapter. They are:

(1) an intrapersonal perspective of pain;
(2) the intrapersonal nature of pain in which we look at the physiology of pain;
(3) interpersonal pain.

As a result the following objectives will be addressed:

- Demonstrate an understanding of the physiological processes involved in the intrapersonal communication of the pain experience.
- Demonstrate an understanding of the role of interpersonal communication on the way pain is perceived in the social and professional context.

Intrapersonal perspective of pain

Although this book is aimed at managing pain, it should be recognized that some pain does have a function and that this function relates to communicating information from within the body and outside of the body to the brain. In this way pain acts as an *intrapersonal* communication mechanism and achieves the following:

- An alarm signal – warning about impending or actual injury or disease;
- Motivation to escape from harm; that is, the thing that is causing the pain;
- Protection of painful or injured area.

These are powerful actions that affect the behaviour of the individual experiencing pain. These drives originate as biologically programmed behaviours in the form of instinctive responses (Main and Spanswick, 2000) but as we grow and develop our behaviours become shaped by personal and social experiences. This idea of functional pain is often associated with acute pain that drives a person to take action; consequently, pains that continue after this, or once help is received, are often viewed as nonfunctional. The motivational effects of the pain however are still exerted on an individual regardless of the functionality of the pain.

Pain is often considered to be a private or intrapersonal experience by individuals who suffer pain and by those who care for them. This concept lies at the heart of many of the problems seen in pain management because, in order to help someone in pain, we need information about their condition. This requires their intrapersonal experience to be translated into an interpersonal experience in order for helping or other actions to occur. Pain is a communal experience that shapes an observer's behaviours and feelings (Goubert et al., 2005) and a communications perspective provides a way for health professionals to reflect on how we respond to the person in pain.

Considering pain from a communication perspective fits nicely within a biopsychosocial model of pain as it maintains a hierarchical systems-oriented approach while providing a rationale for how the different systems interact with each other. It also allows us to focus on pain as a normal functioning system and to explore failure in communications as a dysfunction or pathology in this system. This approach is not meant to replace a standard biomedical approach to pain as a function of the nervous system but to complement it and to add colour in those areas that the biomedical model does not usually consider.

Before we proceed it will be useful to review the

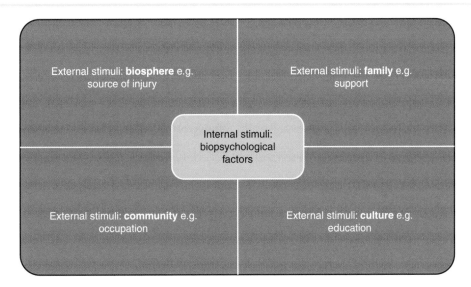

Figure 3.1 The intrapersonal perspective of pain

work you have covered in Chapter 1 on the biopsycho-social model.

Biopsychosocial model and communication

The biopsychosocial model is considered to be a hier-archical model. That is, it is built up of systems – starting at the subatomic and moving up through the physiological systems, to the brain where the *bio* becomes the *psycho* and then out to the wider world away from the individual as we enter the *social* domain. Figure 3.1 sums this up from a communica-tion perspective; external stimuli interact with the body and provoke or are mediated by internal stimuli. This is an intrapersonal perspective of pain. However, this can also be represented from a biopsychosocial perspective.

Although intrapersonal pain largely falls within the remit of the nervous system, a biopsychosocial systems approach can still be applied to it. This can be seen if we start at the lowest level and work upwards to the 'mind' considering different factors that might cause pain at each of the following intrapersonal hierarchical level.

- *Molecular:* one of the neurotransmitters known to provoke a pain response in the nervous system is substance P. Substance P is a neuropeptide; that is, it is a molecule found in the nervous system that is made up of a short chain of proteins. It occurs in the dorsal horn of the spinal cord, as well as other places, and is involved in the transmission of pain from the peripheral nervous system (PNS) to the central nervous system (CNS). It is involved in the pain gate.

- *Genetic:* there are many genetic disorders that produce painful conditions or can lead to insensitivity to pain and subsequent consequences. For example sickle cell, a genetic disorder that affects the shape of red blood cells.

- *Cellular:* when cells are damaged, they release noxious chemicals that stimulate the nervous sys-tem and evoke a pain. We go into this in more detail later in this chapter.

- *Tissue:* an important portion of the nervous sys-tem is the dorsal horn of the spinal cord. This is where the theoretical pain gate is located and inside this region are tissues that contain cells that can modulate pain transmission and either increase or decrease pain.

- *Organ:* almost all our organs can evoke pain; some like the skin are jam-packed with sensors just for this purpose, but there is one organ that is unique. The brain itself does not contain pain receptors, unlike the kidney; for example, it is possible to perform surgery on the brain without any analgesia, just local anaesthetic for the skin. However, in humans the brain is where pain is perceived, it is where meaning is acquired and our emotions impact on our experience of pain. The brain is also where our mind is located. It is here where we perceive ourselves as different to others.

- *Organ systems:* as with organs, many organ systems can be involved in an episode of pain, but without one particular system pain could not be evoked, transmitted or perceived. Among the many jobs that the nervous system does, a normal, healthy functioning nervous system detects and transmits nociceptive pain. When it is unhealthy, if it is damaged in some form then it will produce abnormal pain responses. These arise from within the nervous system and are known as neuropathic pains. This distinction is important if we are to understand the intrapersonal nature of pain.

The intrapersonal nature of pain

We cannot talk about pain communication without discussing the nervous system and its role in detecting pain and transmitting it to the brain. So far we have briefly mentioned two types of pain in connection with the nervous system and pain, nociceptive pain and neuropathic pain. Let us look at these in more depth.

Nociceptive pain

Nociceptive pain can best be described using *gate control theory*. Its underlining principle is that the pain a person perceives is modulated by processes within the nervous system and is not merely a result of the size of the stimulus in relevant neurones as postulated by earlier theories. This explains how factors like mood, thoughts, emotions and past experiences play a role in the actual feeling of pain. It also helps to explain how some peripheral actions, such as rubbing or cold or heat therapies, can help modify pain.

In other words, in gate control theory, pain is regarded as the end result of all these processes and not as the original message from the site of injury. This original message is one input among many conflicting stimuli. To emphasize this we will call the

originating message a **noxious stimulus** and the whole process from detection to perception, nociceptive transmission.

Nociceptive transmission originates in the PNS and is transmitted by an intact and healthy sensory nervous system to the CNS, the brain and spinal cord. It is only in the CNS, particularly within the higher brain centres, that pain occurs because it is here that it is perceived and interpreted and this is the reason why every pain experienced is unique and subjective.

Gate control theory of pain

Ronald Melzack and Patrick Wall first described gate control theory in the early 1960s. They were able to assimilate earlier models of pain with elements that were then hard to explain. Since its development there has been much research into pain and although the original theory has been further developed, it has proven to be robust and provides a useful and practical explanation of our current knowledge of pain. A useful text to explore the theory behind this model and its development and use in practice is Melzack and Wall's book *The Challenge of Pain* (Melzack and Wall, 1996).

The gate control theory of pain involves two stages:

1. Stimuli detection in the sensory nervous system and **modulation** in the spinal cord;
2. Processing and perception of the stimulus as 'pain' in the brain.

Nociceptive transmission

Before we discuss the physiology of nociception we would like you to consider what happens when you stub a toe, a particularly unpleasant event that we are certain all of you will have experienced as this provides a convenient model to explain the process of detection, transmission, modulation and perception.

Activity 3.1

Think back to when you last stubbed a big toe. Describe how the pain felt and what you did after the event.

Physiological response to stubbing your toe	Explanation
A sharp severe pain	Aδ neurone high threshold mechanoreceptors respond to the crush injury Pain seems instant but is actually delayed by a few microseconds Intense pain lasting for several seconds
Instantly pull toe away from the site of injury	A reflex arc response is triggered
Shouting and swearing	The intense initial noxious stimuli ascends to the brain and invokes an emotional response
Feeling nauseous	It also produces a systemic physical response
Hop about and don't attempt to weight-bear	A protective pain behaviour
Grabbing toe and gently squeezing	Again a protective pain behaviour that stimulates the Aβ neurones, producing counter-stimulation and gating
Sharp severe pain eases off, replaced by an aching, throbbing, heavy pain	This indicates C neurone activation Although both Aδ and C neuroreceptors are stimulated at the same time, the relative difference in conduction velocity means that C neurones appear to have a delayed response
New pain increases in intensity over a few minutes and spreads	As a result of an inflammatory response, chemicals released by tissue damage activate other C neurones increasing nociceptive 'noise'
Feeling emotional, irritable and angry	The ascending message has reached the limbic region, arousing an emotional response
Seeking help	A protective behaviour where the intrapersonal becomes interpersonal
The toe feels warm and appears red and swollen	Inflammation heats the surrounding tissue, local temperatures can reach over 40° C and when they do they trigger 'silent' nociceptors to fire
Difficult to weight-bear, walk on your heel	A short-term protective response preventing further tissue damage caused by hyperalgesia
Rubbing or gentle squeezing or application of cold temporarily eases the pain	Because Aβ neurones activity reduce pain gating and ice cools the skin reducing thermoreceptor nociception and inflammation
You may take analgesics	A protective behaviour that artificially inhibits noxious transmission and perception
Over a period of time, hours or more the pain gradually eases	The inflammatory response diminishes as healing occurs

Table 3.1 The physiological response to pain

In Table 3.1 we have listed the sequence of events you should have documented in the order they are likely to occur and we have given a brief description of the physiological process involved.

This sequence of events is common to everyone who hurts themselves through a sudden traumatic injury. Although this example does not take into account individual variation in the pain experience, each stage in this sequence can be related to the various physiological processes that make up a nociceptive transmission.

Detection and modulation

Three sensory nerves are involved in detection and modulation of noxious stimuli, **Aδ (A delta) neurones, C neurones and Aβ (A beta) neurones**. These neurones have different properties that dictate how they act during nociceptive transmission (Table 3.2).

From Table 3.1 we can see that Aδ and C neurones transmit noxious stimuli, these are often referred to as the 'pain neurones' while Aβ neurones transmit non-noxious stimuli. Neurone speed is important in nociceptive transmission and this table shows big differences in conduction velocity. C neurones are by far the slowest (up to 60 times slower than Aδ neurones) because they are thinner and lack a **myelin sheath**. Myelin is a fatty protein that protects, nourishes and insulates the nerve neurones. Aβ neurones are the fastest which means that a stimulus such as gentle squeezing or rubbing can beat a noxious stimulus to the CNS. All three neurones innervate the skin while only C neurones innervate deeper structures such as the gut or joints. Most peripheral nerves are C neurones.

Cutaneous receptors

The skin is packed with sensory apparatus composed of nerve receptors and neurones which are unevenly distributed around the body. In Activity 3.1 you stubbed your toe, damaging soft tissue and stimulating the cutaneous receptors surrounding the toe. These are modified nerve endings, they receive information from outside a neurone and convert this into electrical energy to be propagated, along the neurone, towards the CNS. This process is called **transduction**.

Receptors usually respond to specific types of stimuli and only when the intensity of the stimuli reaches a specific level of intensity or **threshold**. Touch receptors respond to a low threshold of stimuli, while nociceptive receptors generally have a high threshold of stimulation responding to stimuli that damage or have the potential to damage tissue. There are three broad categories of nociceptors:

(1) *High threshold mechanoreceptors:* these respond to mechanical distortion, such as pressure and injury. Structurally simple they are widely distributed and associated with Aδ neurones. It is the first noxious impulse to be experienced after injury and is perceived as sharp, localized or pricking pain.

(2) *Thermal nociceptors:* these respond to particular temperature ranges and supply information about the difference in temperature between the skin surface and the environment. Their threshold is reached when a change in temperature occurs. The quicker the change in temperature the greater the stimulation; this explains why placing icy cold hands into warm water is painful.

Cold receptors are located in the upper layers of the dermis and the epidermis. They are quicker to respond to instant temperature changes than the deeper warmth receptors. Cold receptors are also more numerous than warm receptors. This explains why it is easier to localize a cold sensation and why warm sensations affect a larger area. Within a normal range of temperature, thermoreceptors adapt within to small temperature changes but above 45°C they are non-adapting responding as nociceptive receptors, and above 47°C produce a burning sensation.

(3) *Polymodal receptors* are multifunctional, responding to mechanical and thermal stimuli and also to chemical stimuli. Chemical receptors respond extrinsically to: acids (ant bites); alkalis (bee stings and venom); irritants (capsaicin – from the chilli pepper) and to hypertonic and hypotonic solutions. Internally they are very sensitive to inflammatory processes and are easily destroyed by trauma and chemicals released from damaged tissues. C neurones have polymodal nociceptors and are widely distributed through most tissues. They are characterized by

Type of neurone	C neurones	Aδ neurones	Aβ neurones
Myelinated	Unmyelinated	Myelinated	Myelinated
Diameter	0.2–1 μm	1–6 μm	6–14 μm
Velocity	0.2–1 m/s	12–30 m/s	36–90 m/s
Receptor type	Polymodal nociceptors, hot and cold thermoreceptors, mechanoreceptors	Mechano-nociceptors Cold thermoreceptors Mechanoreceptors	Low threshold Mechanoreceptors Proprioceptors
Stimuli	Chemicals, temperature, movement and pressure	Cold, heavy pressure	Gentle pressure, light touch, proprioception
Noxious stimuli	Slow pain	Fast pain	Non-noxious

Table 3.2 Properties of different sensory nerves

dull, burning and aching pains that may be difficult to localize.

Visceral receptors

Unlike the skin, the organs of the abdomen and thorax are poorly innervated, mainly by C neurones with polymodal receptors. Distribution is not even; some viscera, such as the bronchi, are highly innervated, while others, such as alveoli have a very poor supply. The receptors take three forms:

1. *High threshold receptors:* widely distributed across viscera and only respond to noxious stimuli.
2. *Intensity-coding receptors:* these are less widely distributed, mainly in the heart, oesophagus, colon, urinary bladder and testes. They have a low threshold to natural stimuli and respond to both innocuous and noxious stimuli.
3. *'Silent nociceptors':* making up to a third of visceral receptors and also found in joints they are normally quiet unless an inflammatory process triggers them off.

Inflammation and primary hyperalgesia

Within a few seconds of tissue injury, inflammatory processes are mobilized and these increase nociceptive stimuli in the following ways:

- The neurones themselves may have been damaged and trigger a strong nociceptive signal.
- Damaged cells surrounding the nerves release stimulating chemicals. These trigger C neurone chemoreceptors; they also reduce the threshold at which the receptors activate. This is known as primary hyperalgesia.
- These chemicals trigger an inflammatory response, producing vasodilation, localized heat and releasing histamine and other substances into the tissue.
- These sensitize C neurones making them more likely to fire.
- These chemicals wash around adjacent C neurones, intensifying and spreading pain.
- Rapid localized heat exceeding 40°C which triggers thermoreceptors, adding to the total noxious signal.

Action potentials

Let us think back to our description of the injury to your great toe. The first sensation we described was a strong, intense, sharp pain. This is produced by transmission along the Aδ neurones that terminate in the great toe. This is produced by the high threshold mechanoreceptors of the Aδ neurones as they respond to the increased pressure in their receptive field; in this case the tissue surrounding the big toe caused by the impact of the injury. This intense pain lasts for several seconds or minutes before it is replaced or complemented by other sensations. In neurological terms this is a very long time as one Aδ impulse travelling at 50 metres/second (about the speed of fast car) lasts for a fraction of a second and is acted on by the CNS without us being aware of it. Receptors only propagate the nerve impulse when the stimulus reaches the threshold for that type of receptor. While low threshold receptors respond to different stimuli intensities than high threshold receptors, as long as the threshold is reached a receptor will act regardless of how weak or strong the stimuli is. The biological property behind an impulse is the all-or-nothing **action potential** and these are always of the same intensity. The reasons why we can differentiate between a firm and light stroke are:

- different receptors are stimulated;
- a depolarized receptor produces a **generator potential**. The strength of the stimulus then determines how many subsequent action potentials are propagated. This process of frequency coding is graded; stronger stimuli generate more action potentials per minute than weaker ones. This why despite the refractory period after each action potential a strong stimulus seems to last for longer.
- Another reason is that nociceptors slowly adapt to strong stimuli, whereas weaker stimuli are tuned out as 'background noise', so our nervous system normally ignores touch sensation from our clothing and does not register ambient temperature.
- Finally, nociceptive chemoreceptors are very slow adaptors, so that noxious stimuli from minor wounds, like a paper cut, can persist for hours.

Sensory nerve communication

An impulse is conveyed along neurone axons through electrochemical changes in the cell membrane. This is rapid (See Table 3.2 for difference in conduction velocities) but not instantaneous, although Aδ stimulation might be perceived as such. The impulse then enters the dorsal horn of the spinal cord where:

- Noxious signals carried by Aδ and C neurones and non-noxious signals carried by a Aβ neurones synapse at the dorsal horn, This is where 'pain gating' occurs.

- The strongly graded frequency code of a sudden noxious signal ensures that it is transmitted directly across the spinal cord from the dorsal horn to the ventral horn in a **spinal cord reflex**. Here it synapses with the motor nervous system to automatically move the toe from the source of injury.
- The strong initial nociceptive impulse also travels across the pain gate and up the spinal column to the brain, producing a systemic response before gating activity occurs; this can be emotional and physical.

Key point

Reflex actions occur without any involvement of the brain. We only become aware of them after we have taken the avoiding action. They are actions that protect the body from harm.

The pain gate

This is the site of modulation located in the dorsal horn of the spinal cord, which is the point that all spinal sensory nerves enter the CNS. This is a narrow area and is where the first synapses in the chain of noxious transmission occur. Noxious signals are modulated through conflicting biochemical interactions that occur at neuronal synapses Three factors are involved:

1. The differing characteristics of signals conducted by via C and Aδ and Aβ neurones.
2. Aβ neurones carry innocuous messages about touch and proprioception. These are faster than nociceptive signals; they briefly activate and then inhibit the pain gate. Invoked when you rub your toe a minute or so after the injury occurred, the low-level simulation competes with noxious stimuli, reducing intensity of nociception. It explains how massage works and electrical techniques to manage pain such as **transcutaneous electrical nerve stimulation** (TENS).
3. The first point at which these three neurones terminate. The dorsal horn of the spinal cord is arranged in six layers, or laminae. These contain

neurones that synapse with cells in adjacent laminae. It is here that neurotransmitter activity propagates or modulates the noxious signal. Neurotransmitters that propagate the signal include substance P and **glutamate**. Most nociceptive neurones terminate in the first two outermost laminae; their nociceptive impulse must transfer across several laminae before they can ascend to the brain. β neurones terminate in deeper laminae and thus have a greater impact.

(4) Information arising from modulating factors, such as mood or excitement, exert an influence through descending pathways that also terminate in the dorsal horn. These rely heavily on a group of neurotransmitters known as **endogenous opioid peptides (EOP)**. Opioid drugs mimic the action of EOP.

In the 1960s Melzack and Wall did not know about EOP; they were not discovered for another 10 years. They theorized that there were specific 'transmitter' (T) cells situated in the region of the fifth lamina that were activated or impeded by signals conducted by the sensory nerves. These cells have never been found and it is now believed that the actions in all the lamina cells combine to produce a transmitter/inhibitor effect. The normal state is inhibition; there is constant nociceptive activity inputting to the spinal cord. One example informs us to shift position when we have been sitting still for too long, but most of the time we are unaware of this. It is only when we are bored or wake up in the middle of the night that we may experience mild discomforts that annoy us but which at other times we would not notice.

Descending mechanisms

Modulation at the pain gate was theorized to occur via descending mechanisms that either intensify or inhibit incoming nociceptive messages. There is no physical evidence for such a pathway but the subsequent discovery of several neurotransmitters and their properties explains how modulation occurs.

Neurotransmitters

In the periphery impulses are carried all the way to the dorsal horn by neurones with long axons that only synapse at their terminus. In the brain and dorsal horn, neurones are shorter, and have multi-synaptic connections with adjacent cells. Each synapse requires a neurotransmitter to cross the space for transmission to occur. There are many neurotransmitters involved in nociceptive transmission. These are either excitatory which act to transmit nociception or inhibitory (Table 3.3).

Glutamate is the most abundant excitatory neurotransmitter and like all the other neurotransmitters is not just involved in pain. However, excess glutamate secretion due to intense C neurone activation will stimulate dormant NMDA receptors, sensitize normally quiet spinal neurones and induce cell death in inhibitory neurones, a process known as 'wind-up'. It has been postulated that early intervention can prevent this phenomenon and is the theory behind the action of pre-emptive analgesia.

Secondary hyperalgesia

Under intense continuing stimulation, the initial strong aching sensation transforms into a deep and sickening sensation. This is a sign that activity in the dorsal horn has changed from excitation which amplifies or intensifies noxious signals, to directly affecting the neurones in the dorsal horn, causing them to become more excitable and to form new connections with adjacent cells. This plasticity occurs within a few seconds to several hours after injury and forces you to rest the site of injury and explains what happens in pain after surgery. These changes are usually short lived as healing reduces the tissue damage, lasting several hours or days.

Longer-term plastic changes can also occur as a result of transportation of chemical along C neurones from the site of injury to the dorsal horn of the spinal cord. This is a much slower process than conduction, taking several hours to days but the effect of these chemicals in the dorsal horn is to produce long-lasting changes in noxious transmission. They adversely affect inhibitory mechanisms so that nociception is not diminished and transmission increases. These changes contribute to some of the phenomena seen in chronic pains such as **allodynia** or hypersensitivity to gentle touch.

Neurotransmitter	Action	Receptor	Site
Glutamate	Excitatory	N-methyl-D-aspartate (NMDA), alpha-amino-3-hydroxy-5-methyl-4-isoxazole propionic acid (AMPA) and metabotropic receptors	Widespread in the brain and spinal cord dorsal horn Thalamus Cortex
Substance P	Excitatory	Neurokinin 1 (NK1)	Brain, spinal cord
Neurokinin A and neurokinin B	Excitatory	Neurokinin receptors	Laminae of the dorsal horn
Gamma amino butyric acid (GABA)	Inhibitory	GABA$_A$ GABA$_B$	Widespread in the brain and spinal cord. The interneurones in laminae I, II and III are GABA-rich
Endogenous opioid peptides (EOP)	Inhibitory	mu kappa delta	Cortex, thalamus, dorsal column of the spinal cord, spinal cord laminae
Noradrenalin	Inhibitory	Alpha-2 adrenergic receptor	Throughout the nervous system
Serotonin	Inhibitory in CNS Excitatory in the PNS (an inflammatory product – also in wasp stings and insect venom)	5-HT	Medulla and thalamus, cortex and limbic region

Table 3.3 Properties of neurotransmitters

Ascending pathway

The neurones transmitting sensory information to the spinal cord from the periphery are known as first-order neurones. Once the signal gets through the pain gate they are transferred contralaterally or diagonally to the opposing, ventral side of the spinal cord by second-order neurones. Here they synapse with the lateral **spinothalamic tract** which conveys sensory information on nociception and temperature from every segment of the spinal cord up to the **thalamus** (see Fig. 3.2).

Some of the stranger aspects of pain may arise in the spinothalamic tract; phantom limb pain may be caused by activity in the spinothalamic pathway; strong visceral nociception arriving at one vertebral level may stimulate nociceptive neurones for a different region of the body, leading to referred pain.

The brain

Reticular formation

As the spinothalamic tract enters the brain and terminates at the thalamus, it travels through a complex region of synapses and neurones known as the reticular formation of the hind brain. This is an important

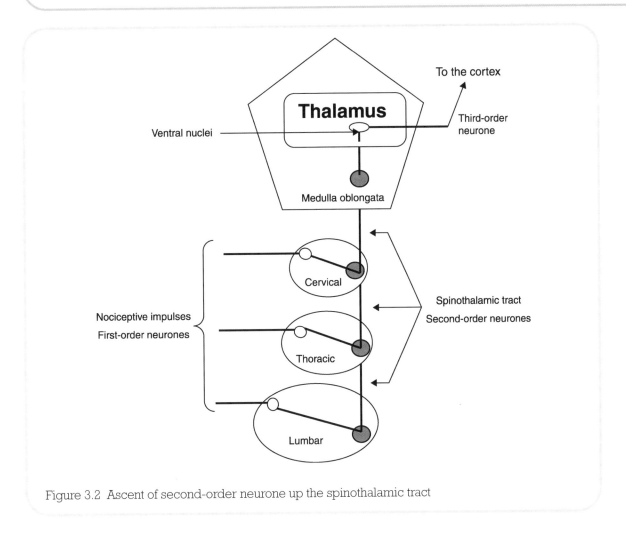

Figure 3.2 Ascent of second-order neurone up the spinothalamic tract

area for modulation of nociceptive impulses. It is also where cranial nerve V, the trigeminal nerve, inputs sensory information from the face.

Thalamus

The thalamus acts as a central switching station where all nociceptive information from the body is processed along with sensory information like touch, proprioception and pressure that have ascended up other pathways. To a large extent our current knowledge of the thalamus's role in pain depends on case history of patients with thalamic lesions and animal experimentation. Newer research, using imaging technology, has added to this and suggests that different regions of the thalamus are involved (Borsook and Becerra, 2006). Modulation and ongoing transmission to the

cortex occurs in the ventral nuclei; the lateral aspect of the thalamus is involved with 'discriminative pain' and the medial aspect with 'affective and motivational' aspects of pain.

Cortex

Third-order neurones, originating in the ventral nuclei of the thalamus (see Fig. 3.2), carry nociceptive information to the cortex. Here we begin to be aware of how nociceptive impulses are modulated and we become aware of them as pain. Imaging techniques demonstrate that the cortex is hierarchically arranged, with the prefrontal cortex at the highest level (Stephenson and Arneric, 2008). Thus:

■ The parietal lobe is involved in the initial awareness of pain and identifying its location.

- The limbic region, one of the earliest parts of the mammalian brain to evolve, is a centre for basic emotional behaviour such as anger. It is involved in the production of EOPs. Here nociception is modulated by emotion.
- The temporal lobe will be involved in pain associated with learning and memory.
- The prefrontal cortex is involved in affective and attention aspects as well as suffering. It used to be thought that it is in this area that pain achieves meaning.

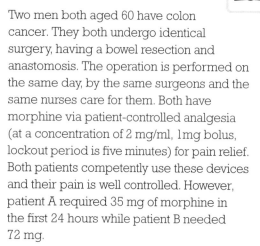

Activity 3.2

Two men both aged 60 have colon cancer. They both undergo identical surgery, having a bowel resection and anastomosis. The operation is performed on the same day, by the same surgeons and the same nurses care for them. Both have morphine via patient-controlled analgesia (at a concentration of 2 mg/ml, 1mg bolus, lockout period is five minutes) for pain relief. Both patients competently use these devices and their pain is well controlled. However, patient A required 35 mg of morphine in the first 24 hours while patient B needed 72 mg.

How does gate control theory help us to understand the differing morphine requirements in these two people with very similar types of injury and disease process? List these in a table.

Differing pain experiences

Gate control theory explains differing pain experiences in individuals with the same injury through considering the effects of modulation. Table 3.4 lists some of the common pain modulating factors seen in surgical pain.

Neuropathic pain

Nociceptive pain arises in a normal healthy nervous system. In our discussion above we have concentrated on acute aspects of nociceptive pain, the commonest

pain and one we have all experienced. An understanding of 'normal' pain is a prerequisite for its management. It also helps to identify pains that fall outside of this parameter. If we confuse nociceptive pain with other types of pain, then we will not provide appropriate treatment and will cause unnecessary suffering.

While nociceptive pains are the commonest form of pain, there are other ways of producing neural signals that are interpreted as pain. There are many pains, like grief, that arise from internal processes and we have already considered how pains can be modified by thoughts, emotions and behaviours. This occurs because each part of the nervous system interacts with all the other parts of the nervous system and in doing so it transforms its physical and chemical structure. In an unhealthy nervous system, one that is damaged or abnormally changed, such interaction produces pains that exhibit different characteristics. We call these 'neuropathic pains' and they tend to:

- Bear no relationship to peripheral stimuli; they may occur without any evidence of external cause;
- Be constant;
- Be associated with sensory changes; innocuous stimuli may provoke pain (allodynia) or sensitivity to stimuli increases (**hyperaesthesia**);
- Be resistant to opioids – demonstrating that normal inhibitory modulation does not work.

Neuropathic pains possess differing characteristics due to their pathology (Table 3.5) and do not respond to the same treatments; consequently, they are much harder to manage.

Characteristics of neuropathic pain

Sensitization

Normally, nociceptors are triggered when a threshold is reached. Inflammatory processes, such as is seen in osteoarthritis, produce chemicals that decrease a receptor's threshold, increasing its sensitivity. This is normal and non-noxious stimuli, like touch, and produce pain. Sometimes inflammation abnormally affects the sympathetic nervous system (SNS). This releases adrenalin and serotonin into the surrounding tissue. In the CNS these produce inhibition but here

Factors which may increase pain	Factors which may diminish pain
Fear or anxiety	Pre-operative information on pain management
Lack of information	Confidence in a good outcome
Fear of anaesthetic	High educational attainment
Past experiences of uncontrolled pain following surgery	Good past experience of pain being managed after surgery
Uncertainty over prognosis; e.g. family member died from bowel cancer	Inclusion in pain assessment process
Low educational attainment	High self-esteem
History of depressive illness	
Existing pain from other sources; e.g. arthritis	

Table 3.4 Common modulation factors after surgery

in the periphery it excites the PNS further reducing the threshold. Even light touch and stimulation we would not normally notice invokes severe pain. Many **neuralgias** exhibit this characteristic.

Abnormal impulses

Abnormal impulses occur when damaged neurones no longer conduct a signal along an axon from the receptor to the synapse; instead the damaged mid-portion of an axon will generate ectopic impulses. A temporary unpleasant example occurs when your *funny bone* is hit or your leg 'falls asleep'. These are characterized by paraesthesia sensation of numbness or *pins and needles*. When damage is permanent the neurone remodels to form ectopic foci; acting as pacemakers these generate repeated signals. These are seen in **neuromas** such as those formed in scar tissue, an example is stump pain. Unlike phantom pain this occurs in a body part that still exists. Neuromas often also exhibit sympathetically mediated sensitization and the resulting pain is characterized as *sharp, burning, electric-like* and *touch-sensitive*. They can also be thermally mediated, with cold worsening the pain and warmth easing it. In some instances it is so severe that wearing a prosthesis is very difficult. Stump pains are also seen following mastectomies, removal of testes and occasionally organs.

Ectopic foci also occur in degenerative diseases of the nervous system such as multiple sclerosis which demyelinize neurones. The result is *hyperexcitability* and spontaneous discharge. When motor nerves are affected twitching and cramp occurs. **Demyelination** also produces crossover of stimuli in adjacent axons, so motor impulses directly produce pain by stimulating nociceptive neurones.

Amplification

Damaged nerves are excited and low-intensity stimuli that would normally never produce pain trigger noxious impulses. As we experience so many low-level stimuli then amplification occurs as nociceptors constantly fire resulting in severe pain that lasts for much longer than the stimulation.

Post-herpetic neuralgia (PHN), a neuropathic pain arising after acute exacerbation of *Herpes zoster* infection (shingles) will persist in over a fifth of people for one month after healing and in a smaller group for many months. It is characterized by amplification and presents as a burning, tingling pain sometimes associated with stabbing sensations which occur along the distribution of usually one, but sometimes more than one, peripheral nerve. The overlying skin may exhibit marked superficial pain with light touch (allodynia) and hyperaesthesia. Curiously,

Type of pain	Nociceptive characteristics	Neuropathic characteristics	Symptom
Osteoarthritis	Inflammatory sensitization Silent nociceptors Wind-up	None	Pain to normal touch
Post-herpetic neuralgia		Sensitization due to sympathetic nervous system (SNS) activity Amplification Abnormal central processing	Allodynia hyperaesthesia
Stump pain	Sensitization due to inflammation	Neuroma formation Sensitization due to SNS activity Hyperexcitability Sympathetically mediated pain (SMP) Trigger points	Sharp, burning, electric shock Touch-sensitive Hyperpathia
Multiple sclerosis	Muscle tension	Ectopic stimuli Hyperexcitability Crossover Central pain	Paraesthesia Twitching and cramp, movement-induced pain Hyperpathia Hyperalgesia
Phantom pain	Wind-up Muscle tension	Crossover Abnormal central processing Loss of $A\beta$ counter-stimulation Response to cold neural reorganization Central pain	Paraesthesia Twitching and cramp, movement-induced pain
Spinal cord lesion pain	Wind-up	Ectopic stimuli Abnormal central processing Loss of $A\beta$ stimulation	Paraesthesia Hyperpathia Hyperalgesia
Fibromyalgia	Nociception	SMP Abnormal central processing Trigger points	Muscle cramps Burning pain Hyperalgesia Trigger points Hyperpathia

Table 3.5 Examples of types and characteristics of different pain

firm pressure may provide pain relief whereas light brushing is unbearable.

Sympathetically maintained pains (SMPs)

The SNS forms part of the autonomic nervous system (ANS) whose actions are largely involuntary in contrast to those of the sensory and motor systems. It predominantly transmits impulses along C neurones from the CNS to organ systems and is involved in the regulation of bodily systems. Occasionally the SNS becomes locally dysfunctional, either due to trauma or some other form of tissue damage resulting in sensitization. Any pain that is sympathetically mediated is exacerbated when the sympathetic nervous system is activated. Psychological reactions that elicit the stress response will contribute to sympathetically mediated pains, thus emotional upset or anger can make pain worse.

SMPs are chronic and are characterized by burning pain. Examples include chronic pancreatitis and pains that involve limbs. They are prone to exacerbation in the winter as temperature affects the ANS, producing hyper-reactive vasomotor response (especially to cold), and colour changes. Secondary changes can be seen due to prolonged SNS overactivity producing oedema, muscle atrophy, bone reabsorption, hair loss and brittle nails.

There are two main types of SMP: complex **regional pain syndrome (CRPS)** Type I or **reflex sympathetic dystrophy** and **CRPS** Type II or **causalgia**.

CRPS Type I initially starts with a trivial injury and usually affects a limb. The sufferer may not even recall the event that caused the pain. Initially, the normal ache and sharp pain of the injury occurs followed by no symptoms for a few weeks to a month or so before the burning pain starts.

CRPS Type II displays the same symptoms but usually follows a traumatic injury such as crush injury, or explosive or bullet wound. It may also occur following surgery. In addition to having abnormal sympathetic activity, there is also a sensory or motor nerve injury with associated muscle control or sensation problems.

All SMPs become entrenched and difficult to treat the longer they are left untreated. Appropriate treatment involves a combination of nerve blocks and intensive physiotherapy; the aim being to restore function while reducing positive feedback caused by the hyperactive SNS. These pains arise outside of the nociceptive nervous system and do not respond to conventional analgesia.

Abnormal central processing

> **Key point**
>
> In neuropathic pains there is too much excitation and insufficient inhibition.

The above neuropathic pains occur because the PNS acts abnormally. However, neuropathic pains also arise when the CNS abnormally processes nociceptive signals or CNS is damaged and abnormally discharges noxious signals.

Functional MRI scans display profound differences in brain activity between nociceptive and neuropathic pain:

- The parietal lobe displays increased activity indicating that the neuropathic pain is perceived as globally affecting the body while nociceptive pains tend to be localized.
- Increased activity in the frontal lobe indicates that pain attention and perception increase, demonstrating the greater influence thought and behaviour has in neuropathic pain. For example, neuropathic pains are associated with more suffering.
- Summation, where brief episodes of intense nociceptive pain produces long-term neuropathic pain and delay of onset can only occur because of central mechanisms.
- Normal wind-up is exacerbated and does not respond to conventional treatments; for example, opioids. This unabated wind-up produces secondary hyperalgesia. Even mild stimulation can elicit and reinforce wind-up and produce an intense pain.

Central pain

Neuropathic pain is also caused by lesions to the CNS when parts of the spinothalamic tract or the brain involved in processing pain are damaged. This type of pain is termed 'central pain'; 8–10 per cent of stroke patients experience moderate to severe symptoms and it is also seen in spinal cord injury, AIDS and multiple sclerosis. Its symptoms are a continuous moderate to severe burning, aching or lacerating sensation affecting a specific region or in some instances the whole body. Cold and light touch applied to the affected area produce a different burning sensation and numbness, decreased temperature sensibility and shooting pains also occur.

The diagnostic burning pain evoked by light touch is probably the worst symptom. It displays slow spatial summation with a delayed onset but, after about 30 seconds, increases in power and severity. It also invokes pain in a much larger area than that stimulated by the initial touch. This means that pain is made worse by rubbing or the touch of clothing. Central pains have been expressed as *indescribable torture*.

Mixed nociceptive/neuropathic pain

Some pains, like fibromyalgia, arise from peripheral nociceptive stimuli but exhibit symptoms such as sleep disorder, fatigue and widespread varying pain that indicate abnormal central processing. Dysfunction in serotonin activity, which modulates sleep as well as pain, may be a contributing factor. This leads to loss of inhibition at neural synapses resulting in acute pain responses that are out of proportion to the insult; for example, **trigger point** stimulation produces an exacerbated response.

Complex pain sensation

Phantom sensations are real phenomena occurring in over 70 per cent of cases following amputation. They do not just affect limbs and have been reported following removal of organs: rectum, vagina, testicles, penis and breasts, in spinal cord injury and in **deafferentation** injuries.

They take three forms:

1. Benign sensations that do not cause distress and may be helpful; for example, with prosthesis management. These include tingling, itching and feeling wet. These make up the majority of phantom sensations.

2. Unpleasant non-pain sensations that cause distress but are not painful. These include: telescoping, as limbs feel like they are shrinking or expanding; awkward positioning or orientation of the phantom limb – as if it were broken or dislocated and penile erection; limb orientation in an unnatural direction. These result in severe cramps and discomfort.

3. Phantom pain, less common than the other two but still a widespread experience. Presenting as burning, shooting, ischaemic or crushing pain, it is often described as similar to and often worse than the pain experienced prior to amputation or surgery.

In phantom sensations the amputated body part still exists in the brain despite changes occurring in the periphery. This suggests that these sensations occur in a normal nervous system and the CNS does not develop abnormal pathology. It originates through intense wind-up and it persists due to the structural changes this produces and ongoing stimulation via the stump and muscular changes as well as loss of $A\beta$ neurone inhibition. Clinically, actions that reduce muscle tension and cramp, such as massage, trigger point injections, visualization and stretching, which seem to ease phantom sensations, might support this theory although there are probably structural changes in the brain as well.

Interpersonal pain

Humans are a social organism and pain is experienced within the social sphere that humans live in. It has been described as a fundamental social event (Craig, 2003) that influences individuals, the family and wider aspects of society from birth to death. Indeed, there is increasing evidence that pain may be experienced by the fetus so that it exerts an influence before birth occurs. Pain is therefore a prime shaper of our physical experiences, our psychological experiences and our social experiences. Craig (2003) suggests that a broader interpersonal model is required if we wish to explore how interactions with others shapes our experiences of pain (Fig. 3.3).

From this perspective pain is not a private experience it:

- signals danger to others;
- elicits sympathy in others;

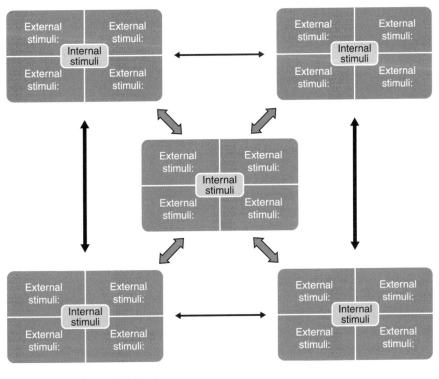

Figure 3.3 Interpersonal model of pain

- instigates empathy and a desire to help in others;
- influences communal bonds.

Pain is therefore at least partially a public event. It is intimately associated with motor behaviours but these behaviours become modified by social codes of acceptable and allowable behaviour.

Activity 3.3

When we are on our own and experience pain we may display very different behaviours than when we are in the presence of others. We might also display different behaviours in front of different people. Each reaction is a genuine response to the pain but the display will vary. Think about your pain behaviours? Compare the differences that occur in front of the following people. For example would you be more or less likely to shout, swear or cry, go quiet, avoid company, seek help, protect the injured area in the following situations:

- on your own;
- with your partner;
- with your mother;
- with other family members;
- with friends;
- with work colleagues;
- with strangers.

Influences on pain responses

Key point

The key to interpersonal communication with someone in pain is active listening. This involves more than hearing words; it requires reading verbal and non-verbal cues, an attitude of respect and acceptance, and a willingness to see things from another's perspective.

It is important to realize that pain responses vary between individuals. When alone you may be quite loud and expressive; you may shout and swear if you hit yourself with a hammer. Alternatively, you may be fairly stoical in your response and may just wince, shake your injured thumb and carry on with the job.

Responses with partners also vary greatly and depend on several factors: the openness of the relationship; how supportive your partner is to your emotional needs; how perceptive they are at recognizing and acting on cues for action from your behaviour; the relationship's normal emotional display rules; whether the pain is acute or chronic and the perception of honesty in the pain display.

The interrelation between people in pain and partners and also with others is a rich area for cognitive and behavioural research. An interesting model is the community coping model (CCM) (Thorne et al., 2004). This model theorizes that people in pain communicate their pain experience in order to gather social proximity and support with the intention of reducing distress rather than reducing pain (Sullivan et al., 2006).

Children's pain responses to mothers depend on the emotional dynamics between mother and child and also on age. In a very young child the immediate response to pain is for the child to look at their mother (Main and Spanswick, 2000). Awareness that someone else is experiencing pain is an event that can be of profound importance because it acts as a command for their attention. It provokes vicarious fear for personal safety of the onlooker and their kin. In other words, are they or their children in danger from the cause of the pain?

Responses to other family members depends on the nature of your relationship with them; siblings commonly compete with each other, leading to either demonstrations of greater stoicism, in order to diminish pain behaviours or exaggeration in order to draw more attention. These patterns are often established in childhood as a consequence of seeking parental support and attention and persist into adulthood. Some relationships may be heavily gender influenced; for example, the relationship between a father and a daughter can be qualitatively different than that between a father and son. Such roles may enforce social expectations of how a woman or a man is expected to behave when in pain.

With friends your behaviour may depend on your level of intimacy with them. Some friends can be close confidants and a strong source of social support. Others you may feel are less likely to be supportive and may be driven away by an overt display of pain behaviours.

Work colleagues may also vary in their responses. Some will be considerate, demonstrating empathy and concern while others may only be concerned about the impact on their workload. Such peer pressure might cause you to carry on working despite the pain. If this is the case you would be likely to mask behavioural displays.

When in the presence of strangers, social controls are often at their strongest and pain acts as a barrier to communication. Unless the pain is so severe that they cannot function, it is unlikely that someone will display their pain. However, when in severe pain, people ignore normal rules of social exchange as they seek help. Responses to these appeals are coloured by their pain experience and they become hypersensitive to actions and attitudes and interpret responses to their pain as a judgement about their worth. At the same time they become insensitive to others' needs as they focus on conveying their problems to elicit help and concern from others.

This preoccupation with their pain influences the attitudes and behaviours of others towards people in pain. This is a normal response and is shaped by context and experience. A display of empathy is more in certain environments (Goubert et al., 2005) or if we are satisfied with the 'truthfulness' of their pain (Sullivan et al., 2006).

Pain displays also indicate social capacity to function. If it is an acute pain, the onlooker wants to know how severe it is, do they just need to rest, or do they need to seek professional help? If the pain is chronic pain are they still able to contribute to communal social well-being or will they be a drain on the resources of those around them? Chronic pains are often subject to stricter social regulation, such as toleration of pain signals because of this impact on others. Pain has a substantial impact on social relations and security. It can affect bonding relationships between partners and has an effect on development in children.

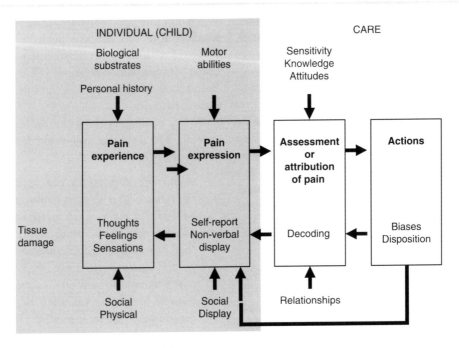

Figure 3.4 Sociocommunication model
Source: adapted from Craig (2003)

A sociocommunication model of pain

Craig (2003) describes a complex model of communi-cation of pain as seen in Fig. 3.4. This model origin-ated from work done with children but we have extrapolated the principles to any person.

The model relies on a series of interacting dimen-sions, the personal experience of pain, its expression, how others respond to this expression and the actions they take and biases they hold or develop as a result of interacting with the person in pain. Each dimension builds on and shapes those they interact with.

The pain experience

This first dimension considers the total pain experi-ence. It represents the physical, social and psycho-logical dimension of the intrapersonal experience of pain. This pain experience is originally biologically programmed behaviour in the form of instinctive responses (Main and Spanswick, 2000) but as we develop our behaviours become shaped by social interactions and learning processes. These modify our expression of pain.

Expression of pain

The second dimension depends on the ability of the person in pain to communicate and move within the realms of social rules that govern pain display; they are also heavily influenced by the actions and reac-tions of those around us. This expression communi-cates our pain experience to others.

Assessment or attribution of pain

The ability to understand pain expression is shaped by a range of factors including knowledge and the rela-tionship of the carer to the person in pain. These fac-tors will predispose them to take action.

Actions

Carers may take action to help but ignore the pain. They might avoid contact because they are distressed or because they do not know how to handle the pain. They might also make the wrong supporting measure and make the pain worse. Actions will depend on biases and dispositions the carer holds.

The effect of this action has consequences for future dealings between the person in pain and their carer and may well shape responses to similar carers. If the person is a nurse and is found to be unsympathetic then the assumption may be made that all nurses will behave in this way creating dissatisfaction as well as increasing distress.

When caring for people in pain we need to be aware of the influences of their pain behaviours on how we respond to them. If we can understand the way people communicate their pain and how this prompts our colleagues and ourselves to respond, then we can identify where we need to moderate our behaviours and responses in order to reduce distress.

The language of pain

To health professionals pain is a very important symptom in any field of medicine. As a result there has developed a wide vocabulary of words to describe the symptoms of pain and discomfort. There are lots of technical words to describe pain; for example, causalgia, hyperalgesia, allodynia, dysthaesia and neuralgia, neuritis, but putting them into layman's terms is not easy. The technical descriptors mean specific things to an expert and have been written in glossaries such as the one prepared for the International Association for Study of Pain by Merskey and Bogduk (1994). The International Association for Study of Pain's website offers a version of this glossary and if you access it you can see that it is clearly meant to provide descriptors for those already familiar with the terms. For example:

Causalgia
A syndrome of sustained burning pain, allodynia, and hyperpathia after a traumatic nerve lesion, often combined with vasomotor and sudomotor dysfunction and later trophic changes.

(Merskey and Bogduk, 1994)

It is clear that this description would not be suitable for any but the most well-indoctrinated patient or client, perhaps another doctor! They have been described because there was a need for a common language of pain among professionals. This need is so important that proposed recent changes to update this terminology (Loeser and Treede, 2008) require careful negotiation and provoke a flurry of responses. In other words, before this list was published there was a chance of confusion and uncertainty in the communication between fellow specialists. In fact, you probably had to look up various descriptions in order to complete the activity.

We try to simplify things for our patients and clients and it is likely that you would describe causalgia as something like:

A burning pain which can be produced by light touch that does not normally produce pain and is made much worse when repeatedly touched, all of which occurs in an area that has been damaged following injury or surgery when a nerve was severed or otherwise damaged and is accompanied by changes in the surrounding tissue such as muscle wasting and unusual responses to heat or cold.

This is of course only an approximation of the actual technical descriptor and even so is long winded and difficult to follow. Even when put into simpler terms, it would still not be suitable for many people; how about interpreting this for a child, or someone with a learning disability?

We can of course make things easier; for example, if we take just the simple descriptors for intensity of pain (no pain, mild, moderate, severe) we might assume that these provide an adequate explanation of how bad the pain is for our patients or clients but once again they are just an approximation. This is probably fine if you have a good idea of what is causing the pain, but that depends on you making the assumption that you do know what is causing the pain. For example, it might seem reasonable to assume that pain after surgery for a hip replacement is located in the region of the arthroplasty but what if it is present because of pain in the lower back, perhaps as a consequence of the surgery or perhaps as an exacerbation of an ongoing problem. Simple explanations by their nature lose detail and this detail might well be necessary for true understanding.

Essentially, what we are doing is attempting to map out the relationship between a private experience (pain) and the expression of that private experience (in language) (Smith, 1998). This is problematic at the best of times and may well be very contentious.

> *When the experience cannot be shared, our reliance on the shared 'meanings' of words is complete. This is of course true of communication in general but for many uses of everyday language there are both linguistic and non-linguistic opportunities to ascertain that meaning is shared or, if it is not shared, to establish understanding.*
>
> (Smith, 1998: 28)

What Smith (1998) tells us is language normally develops through shared, everyday experiences and events like pain, which are internal and private, are usually not an everyday experience. Even when it is an everyday experience, the frustration of getting others to understand it or even to listen to it gets in the way of expression. In other words, there is a lot of room for misunderstanding when a health professional tries to understand the pain someone is experiencing. In Chapter 4 on assessment of pain, we address how we can attempt to overcome these problems. For now you have to realize that when you ask someone about their pain there is a high probability that you will be mistaken in your interpretation of their problem unless you are very careful.

Something lost in the translation

We really have several different languages of pain. There is one that health professionals with an interest in pain are familiar with and with which you by reading this book are becoming familiar. This attempts to codify pain in a scientific and technical sense in order to understand it and to communicate this understanding to other professionals. There is another which is the personal expression of an experience of pain, a language we also make use of when we are in pain but one that is based on internal processes and has to be put into words to make others understand. This of course depends on our ability to express ourselves and this involves all sorts of factors including age and education but overlying this is interference of the agony of the pain. Falling between these is a form of pidgin pain language, one that is used to try and interpret the pain experience and fit it

into the technical language and one that if it is too inflexible will fail to do this.

This last form of language makes use of words such as burning, crushing and stabbing although these are adjectives that describe certain actions. They are applied to various pains which are not associated with the action. Unless you have been burnt, crushed or stabbed when you use these words, you are actually imagining what it would be like to experience this. Your understanding will only be as good as your imagination and as good as the imagination of the person you are talking to. You might actually imagine something radically different. Think about when you read a book and then watch a film of the book. How many times have you been disappointed that the film does not live up to your expectations? What you are actually disappointed in is the differences in imagination between the director of the film and you. It is entirely possible that there is a danger of such an event every time we try and understand someone's experiences.

Iatrogenic communication

Failure to communicate can make pain worse (Main and Spanswick, 2000). Not interpreting or understanding clinical findings because of poor comprehension of a verbal description of the pain can result in:

- using an inappropriate treatment that will fail to relieve the pain and may leave the patient with untoward consequences such as addiction to opioids;
- further investigations, perhaps expensive, uncomfortable and unnecessary and onward referral to a different speciality or no further offer of assistance.

Where the carer's body language and verbal language do not match, the message that the pain is *in the mind*, implying it is not real, can be sent. This can result in demands for a second opinion, loss of faith in orthodox medicine and turning to alternative therapies which have dubious evidence of effectiveness and depression, anger or anxiety because there is no one else to turn to. Sometimes communicating with the best intentions can produce adverse effects. Attempting to explain complex problems simply can result in misunderstanding and mistaken beliefs through inappropriate language. For example:

- a scan shows degenerative changes although this is a normal process of ageing and most people would show similar changes;
- someone who is told their spine is 'crumbly' does not dare move as they image their backbone is like a packet of digestive biscuits.

Key point

How you respond to someone is important; even casual remarks can take on great significance and have unintended consequences.

Summary

This chapter has focused on an extremely important aspect of pain management. Communication of the pain experience is crucial to the way we assess, plan, implement and evaluate care.

We have considered communication from two perspectives – intrapersonal and interpersonal. Intrapersonal communication has focused on the way pain is communicated within our bodies. We have explored the physiological processes which enable this communication.

Interpersonal communication examined the way the pain experience is communicated to the outside world and here we have emphasized interrelationship between the individual's experience and expression of pain and the care giver's or recipient's assessment of the message and the resulting actions.

Understanding these two communication processes are important and so we encourage you to extend your reading on these topics.

Reflective activity

As a conclusion to this chapter consider how knowledge of this theory will help you in your future nursing practice. Use this reflective activity to explore your own knowledge, skills and attitudes specifically in relation to the communication of the pain experience. You may like to focus on an experience from practice which illustrates challenges you have faced with respect to the intrapersonal and interpersonal communication of pain or restrict your reflection to an experience that proved challenging from an interpersonal perspective.

Try to be specific and use the following points/questions as a guide:

- *State* which elements of the chapter will help you in your future practice.
- *Elaborate:* be specific in terms of how this knowledge and understanding can be used in practice.
- *Give examples* of care events which would benefit from what you have learnt.
- What are the *implications* if you change the way you practice?

You may prefer to use a reflective model such as Gibbs's (1988) to guide your reflection. See the Appendix at the end of this book. Think of a specific example as the starting point. Describe the event and then proceed through the cycle. When analysing the situation draw on this chapter's theory to support your discussion and demonstrate your understanding. For example, you may like to draw on a personal or professional experience of pain. Consider the intrapersonal communication of the pain in terms of its pathophysiology and reflect on the way you communicated this experience to others, or how others communicate the experience to you. Try to identify your strengths and limitations with respect to your understanding of the physiological processes involved and how better you can communicate with others.

References

Borsook, D. and Becerra, L.R. (2006) Breaking down the barriers: fMRI applications in pain, analgesia and analgesics, *Molecular Pain*, 2(30). Available online at www.ukpmc.ac.uk/classic/picrender.cgi?artid=763732&blobtype=pdf.

Craig, K.D. (2003) The faces of pain: an interpersonal core, paper presented at the Plenary Session V, *Annual Scientific Meeting*, London: The British Pain Society.

Gibbs, G. (1988) *Learning by Doing: A Guide to Teaching and Learning Methods*. Oxford: Further Education Unit, Oxford Polytechnic.

Goubert, L., Craig, K.D., Vervoort, T., Morley, S., Sullivan, M.J.L., Williams, A.C.d.C., Cano, A. and Crombez, G. (2005) Facing others in pain: the effects of empathy, *Pain*, 118(3): 285–88.

Loeser, J.D. and Treede, R.-D. (2008) The Kyoto protocol of IASP basic pain terminology, *Pain*, 137(3): 473–77.

Main, C.J. and Spanswick, C.J. (2000) *Pain Management: An Interdisciplinary Approach*. London: Churchill Livingstone.

Melzack, R. and Wall P.D. (2006) *The Challenge of Pain*, rev. 2nd edn. London: Penguin Books.

Merskey, H. and Bogduk, N. (1994) (ed.) *Classification of Chronic Pain*, 2nd edn. International Association for the Study of Pain Task Force on Taxonomy. Seattle WA, IASP Press. pp. 209–14. Available online at www.iasp-pain.org/AM/Template.cfm?Section=Pain_Definitions&Template=/CM/HTMLDisplay.cfm&ContentID=1728#Causalgia (accessed 25 June 2009).

Smith M.V., (1998) Talking about pain, in B. Carter (ed.) *Perspectives on Pain: Mapping the Territory* (Chapter 3). London: Arnold.

Stephenson, D.T. and Arneric, S.P. (2008) Neuroimaging of pain: advances and future prospects, *The Journal of Pain*, 9(7): 567–79.

Sullivan, M.J.L., Martel, M.O., Tripp, D., Savard, A. and Crombez, G. (2006) The relation between catastrophizing and the communication of pain experience, *Pain*, 122(3): 282–8.

Thorne, B.E., Keefe, F.J. and Anderson, T. (2004) The communal coping model and interpersonal context: problems or process? *Pain*, 110(3): 505–7.

Pain assessment

4

Chapter contents

Introduction

Pain assessment

Assessment as part of care planning

Problems associated with pain assessment

The pain management process

    Factors that influence the experience of pain
        and pain assessment

    Anxiety

    Perceived loss of control

Why assess acute pain?

    How often should acute pain be assessed?

    When should pain be assessed?

    How should acute pain be assessed?

Pain assessment tools

    Subjective measurements

    Verbal rating scales

    VAS

    NRS

    Effectiveness of pain assessment

Pain assessment in children

The assessment of chronic pain

    The process of assessment in chronic
        nonmalignant pain

The character of pain

    Location

    Description

    Time-related factors

    Intensity

    Influencing factors

Psychosocial assessment

Functional assessment

Pain history assessment

Questionnaire methods

Pain diaries and journals

Chronic pain assessment in children

Summary

Reflective activity

References

Further reading

Introduction

One of the fundamental nursing activities related to pain management is the assessment of pain. Much has been written about pain assessment and if you use those two words as a search term in any literature search engine, you will generate a list of references running into tens of thousands. We summarize some of this literature and discuss the properties of some of the more commonly used pain assessment tools that are available; but we are also going to challenge you to consider why pain assessment is so important.

This chapter explores the importance of pain assessment in a variety of pain situations. When discussing acute pain assessment the focus will be on assessment of pain after surgery because this has been recognized as an important area for development of practice and it has seen the biggest investment of resources. It should be stated however that the principles of acute pain assessment outlined here are of value in many different situations. The principles of pain assessment in patients experiencing chronic pain has focused on the influences of the physiological, psychological and sociological aspects of chronic conditions, and the impact these have on the individual expression of pain.

The areas that are covered in this chapter are:

1. factors that influence the experience of pain and pain assessment;
2. where, how and why pain should be assessed;
3. the process of acute and chronic pain assessment in adults and in children and barriers to assessment.

As a result the following objectives will be addressed:

- Demonstrate an awareness of the benefits of acute pain assessment for the care of the person in acute pain.
- Appreciate how an understanding of these benefits can contribute to the avoidance of health problems and complications in people with acute pain, particularly after surgery.
- Evaluate different methods of assessing acute pain.
- Demonstrate an understanding of the physical, psychological and sociological effects of chronic pain.
- Appreciate how an understanding of these elements is vital in order to undertake holistic, effective pain assessment in chronic nonmalignant pain.
- Identify different methods of assessing chronic pain.
- Apply at least one method of chronic pain assessment to practice.

Pain assessment

Pain and discomfort are the most frequent reasons why an individual contacts the health service and failure to assess pain is a major contributor to the inadequacies in pain management. Before we proceed, we must be sure we know what *assessment* actually means. According to Fordham and Dunn (1994: 57), assessment *'is a process by which we come to some conclusion about the nature of a problem'*.

The skills necessary are those of partnership, communication and interpretation of both words and behaviour noticing, observing, validating and verifying our belief in the pain.

Fordham and Dunn (1994) stated briefly the *who, how, what* and *when* approach to assessment:

- *Who* should assess – is the patient, unless patient and nurse do not share a common language, they are unconscious or inarticulate.
- *How* should we assess – by observation, measurement, conversation and recording? 'Tools' that are used to record and transmit information can achieve measurement.
- *What* should we assess – the nature, intensity and site of pain, likely causes, and precipitating factors? In addition, pain's meaning and signifi-

cance to the patient, their coping strategies and desired goal.

- *When* should we assess – regularly, repeatedly – at the request of the patient, in response to the severity of the pain, when pain is expected or anticipated and in order to establish effectiveness. (Fordham and Dunn, 1994; Regnard and Tempest, 1998).

We would like to add one more 'W' word to this list, 'why'. It is extremely important in pain assessment but in our experience is often overlooked.

- *Why* should we assess pain? There are many reasons why pain should be assessed, however, and when we have asked students and others why they want to assess someone's pain, we inevitably get an answer along the lines of 'it's not right to leave someone in pain' or 'it's inhumane' (Hunter, 2000). There are other reasons. In research studies we might want to assess pain because we want to find out something about people's responses to being in pain or more commonly to test how effective a pain treatment is. These are all good reasons; however, we also want you to critically think about why you are going to assess someone's pain within the context of your own practice.

Assessment as part of care planning

In clinical practice, assessment is the first part of a process of treating someone's problem. Once we have made an assessment we can then plan what to do, implement that plan or treatment and then evaluate that plan. If we are going to assess someone's pain then it should be in order to devise and implement a treatment for that pain. If we do this then we should use the same assessment method to evaluate the pain as we used to decide our actions and when we do that we are not only measuring how much pain someone is in, we are also evaluating the intervention and our plan and this means that we are finding out something about the quality of care we deliver.

> **Key point**
>
> Pain assessment is a measure of the quality of our care; it provides information on how good we are at managing someone's pain.

Problems associated with pain assessment

Some of the reasons that make pain difficult to assess are based on the assumptions and misconceptions that both patients/clients and their families on one hand and health care professionals on the other hand may have regarding the assessment and treatment of patients with pain. Such misconceptions include:

1 *Beliefs about who knows the most about the pain:* a common error is that the person who is actually experiencing the pain, that is, the patient, believes that the health care professional is an expert in their pain because they have a wide range of experience in caring for people with their particular problem. However, often this is not the case, as experts in a particular area of health care, such as cardiac pain or a particular type of surgery, often have misplaced ideas about pain threshold and tolerance.

a) *Misplaced ideas about pain threshold:* there is a tendency among health professionals to assume that people with a particular condition experience a uniform response to their pain. This ignores the highly variable reaction often seen as a consequence of variations in tolerance and behavioural and physiological responses to pain.

b) *Pain tolerance* varies greatly between people and in one individual may vary over time. Factors that reduce tolerance include existence of a chronic pain, more than one source of pain, lack of sleep, high levels anxiety and a loss of control. We may see higher levels of tolerance when a person has low anxiety, good social and psychological support mechanisms and a high **locus of control**. As you can see many of these factors may be outside of the individual's control; however, often health care professionals form judgements about a patient or client or their families based on their toleration of pain.

2 *Patients' knowledge of clinicians' expectations of pain behaviours:* people often assume they should behave in a certain way when in pain. These beliefs are shaped by the need to seek help in the form of expressing overt pain behaviours but are often moderated by social norms; for example, men may display pain in a different way to women. Failure to comply with these norms may lead to a person's pain being perceived as false or to concealing pain from health professionals.

3 *Attribution of cause:* often patients/clients and their families may attribute different causes for their pain than health care professionals. This might arise if they have a particular anxiety; for example, that their pain is a sign of a bad prognosis, or because health care professionals may focus on one particular element, their surgical problem for example, and not be aware that the patient may have other pain problems.

4 *Addiction:* a very common concern among patients and clients but also among health professionals is related to the analgesia required for treating severe acute pain. Patients fear that they could become addicted if they take opioids and health care professionals may read someone's

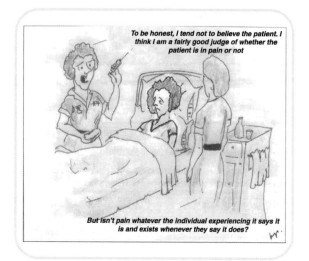

To be honest, I tend not to believe the patient. I think I am a fairly good judge of whether the patient is in pain or not

But isn't pain whatever the individual experiencing it says it is and exists whenever they say it does?

pain behaviour as being a demand for opioids to feed an addiction. This can be a particular problem if the patient's behaviour is already viewed suspiciously: that is, their pain is believed to be less than is reported or is nonexistent.

5. *Placebos:* a person in pain may be utilizing a method of controlling their pain that appears to have no basis in scientific evidence and yet they appear to be getting a benefit from this. This may be due to the **placebo effect**. Consequently, they may be using an inappropriate or even harmful method or may fail to seek help from an appropriate source. Placebos may also be considered by some health professionals as a useful method of dealing with pain where they do not believe the person is in pain, or where they feel they cannot do anything else for the person in pain. Often this is justified on the grounds that they are doing no harm; however, in the first example, they are in weak ethical territory because they are overriding the person's expression of their autonomy. In the second instance, they may be either denying the patient the opportunity to seek help from somewhere else or they may be offering false hope.

The pain management process

Acute pain management is more than a collection of interventions. It is a package of care that needs to be examined as a whole as well as in its parts

(McQuay and Moore, 1998). Pain assessment should be viewed as the starting point of this package of care, a unique role carried out by the multidisciplinary team.

The problem-solving approach adopted by this process involves four stages: assessment (identification of pain), planning (setting a target, e.g., reduce pain to at least a severity score of 3 on a numerical rating scale), implementing the plan (treating the pain) and evaluation of the plan (how effective have we been). The pain management process then begins again with reassessment of the problem. Fordham and Dunn (1994) suggest that problem-solving, beginning with the initial assessment and sustained through regular review and evaluation of treatment, is one of the main principles of effective pain management.

The Joint Report (Royal College of Surgeons and College of Anaesthetists, 1990) on pain after surgery recommended that patients should be involved whenever possible in the systematic assessment of their pain and that this assessment should be recorded.

Ten years later the Clinical Standards Advisory Group on services for patients with pain (CSAG, 2000: 69) made a similar recommendation: '*Institute a standardised approach to the assessment of post-operative and other acute pain throughout . . .*'

The need for CSAG to write a second statement that is essentially the same as the Royal College's Report written 10 years earlier is an indication of concern about the lack of progress in this area and Powell et al. (2009) continue to identify organizational factors as a barrier to achieving this. In a thought-provoking article Carr (2007) points out that difficulties arise when no one person is held accountable for pain management. She asks us to consider the following:

Reflect for a moment on who is accountable in your area: the surgeon? anaesthetist? acute pain team? registrar? the nurse or the patient? Often it is difficult to determine exactly who is accountable as that person may change during the course of the patient's journey. Clear lines of accountability and the communication of these are important aspects of pain management. Personally I

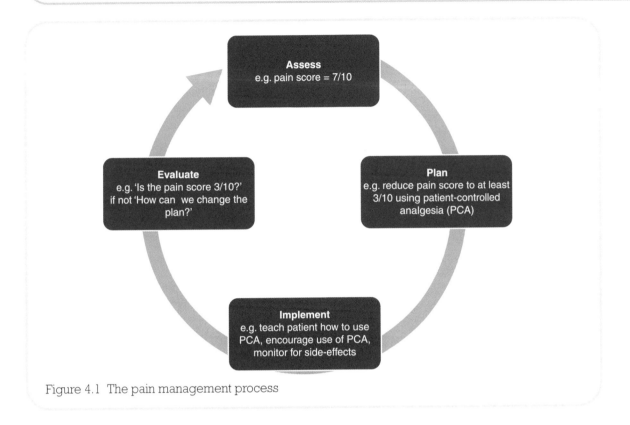

Figure 4.1 The pain management process

view the nurse as being accountable, for he or she is with the patient around the clock and is potentially in the most prominent position to influence the care for the patient.

(Carr, 2007: 200–8)

Key point

Effective pain management will not occur unless someone is held to be accountable.

Factors that influence the experience of pain and pain assessment

It is generally thought that the intensity of the injury response is proportional to the degree of tissue trauma (Chernow, 1987). For example, X operation causes Y amount of tissue damage leading to Z amount of pain and therefore needing N amount of analgesia. Recent research demonstrates that statements X and Y are correct as certain operations pro-

duce more tissue damage than others (Giannoudis et al., 2006), and this is related to the degree of pain experienced (Squirrell et al., 1998) and the type of pain intervention needed to reduce surgical stress (Giannoudis et al., 2006). However, there is no evidence that suggests two people having identical operations should experience the same severity of pain, although other characteristics of their pain are similar. Yet often we hear comparisons between patients who have had similar types of surgery which make links between their ability to tolerate pain and some aspect of their general character. Brockopp et al. (2004) demonstrated in their study that most nurses used information other than the patient's pain when making decisions about pain management and that preconceived notions related to diagnosis, age and gender negatively affected patient care, regardless of the degree of pain experienced by patients.

This is contrary to Melzack and Walls' (1965) theory of pain suggesting that the amount and quality of pain perceived is determined by physiological, psychological, cognitive and emotional variables; that is, pain is a biopsychosocial phenomenon.

Some of the impacts you may have thought of regarding the patient's pain assessment may include reluctance to involve the patient in their pain assessment or disbelief of their pain assessment. This may lead to inaccurate recording of the pain score which may result in inadequate analgesia and the persistence/recurrence of the pain. As a result a vicious circle of pain, disbelief and inadequate analgesia evolves. Alternatively, the patient having expressed their pain during pain assessment and been disbelieved or given inadequate analgesia may cease to complain of pain preferring to put up with the pain rather than 'bother the staff'. Either scenario suggests a failure in the quality of pain management and will impact on the patient's experience and future experience of pain.

According to the Joint Report (Royal College of Surgeons and College of Anaesthetists, 1990) inaccuracies with pain assessment occurred because subjective assessments of pain were being made by staff rather than the patient. However, the literature suggests that nurses are well aware that the authority on the pain is the patient (Watt-Watson, 1987; Brunier et al., 1995; Clarke et al., 1996) even though this knowledge does not seem to be applied in practice (Sloman et al., 2005).

Other studies have consistently highlighted discrepancies between nurses' and patients' assessments of pain over time (Seers, 1987; Schafheutle et al., 2001; Solomon, 2001); and that assessment is strongly influenced by visual cues such as facial expression (Hirsh and Jensen, 2009) and other behaviours displayed by patients (Hamers et al., 1994; Allcock, 1996; Schafheutle et al., 2001) or by assumptions about demographic characteristics, such as age and gender (Brockopp et al., 2004).

However, it must be recognized that some patients do not always express their pain (Defrin et

al., 2006) and may even deny it exists, contributing to any inadequacies in pain assessment and management. Reasons for this include fears about developing opioid tolerance and side-effects, distracting health care professionals from treating their disease and wanting to be a good patient (Tzeng et al., 2006). Although the basic principle is that the individual should make the assessment of their pain, health care professionals within the multidisciplinary team must be familiar with patient-centred barriers to achieve this end.

Some of the things you might have thought about may have included those suggested by Warfield and Stein (1991) who state that:

> in attempting to understand the patient's complaint, a comprehension of factors that influence the perception as well as the cause of pain is essential. Learned behaviour; ethnic, religious, and cultural factors; the context of the painful situation; social influences; and psychological factors all contribute to the complexity of pain perception.
>
> (Warfield and Stein, 1991: 16)

Since pain is a biopsychosocial phenomenon and is subjective, it is important to bear these factors in mind when assessing the patient's pain as we cannot make assumptions on how much pain another person is feeling. Other determinants that may positively or negatively influence the experience of pain include anxiety and perceived control over the pain. While these psychosocial factors may be less readily observable, they are no less harmful and interact with the physical alterations as part of the pain experience.

Anxiety

Anxiety and fear are common emotions accompanying pain. A report by the Audit Commission (1997) suggested that many patients are anxious before their operation and the patient needs information about what is going to happen to them in order to reduce their fears. The type of worries the pre-operative patient has includes the anaesthetic and after-effects of the operation such as pain and nausea (Audit Commission, 1997). In addition, there is evidence that patients worry about other issues as well including distracting health professionals from their job in treating the problem, a fear of injections and worry about being unpopular if they complain (Carr, 2007).

The National Health and Medical Research Council (NHMRC) (1998) state that pain, anxiety and sleeplessness make up a vicious cycle, each aspect influencing the other; that is, anxiety can influence the pain and vice versa. This confirms early findings by Baylock (1968) who suggested that pre-operative anxiety can increase post-operative pain and Closs et al. (1997) who established a link between high anxiety, severe pain and lack of sleep after orthopaedic surgery (Fig. 4.2).

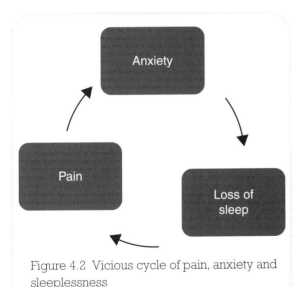

Figure 4.2 Vicious cycle of pain, anxiety and sleeplessness
Source: adapted from NHMRC (1998)

This suggests that as health care professionals we should be preparing patients before an operation or painful procedure by giving them information to reduce anxiety and pain. This preparation includes an explanation of the acute pain assessment chart to be used as well as a warning that unrelieved pain can cause harm (Carr, 2007).

The Audit Commission (1997) survey showed that half of patients remembered talking to an anaesthetist, surgeon and nurse about pain control before an operation, underpinning the importance of all three members of the multidisciplinary team giving consistent advice. They recognized that patients needed an opportunity to discuss the anaesthetist's proposals (for the anaesthetic and analgesia) pre-operatively because unexpected events in the post-operative period cause more distress. Carr (2007) reinforces the need to apply a multidisciplinary approach to such information giving.

From survey information, the Audit Commission recommended a policy for pre-operative information given to patients including both verbal and written information and stress effective collaboration between nursing and medical staff on this issue. According to Salmon (1994), however, the effect of information on individuals differs and what may benefit one patient may harm another. Information that focuses on preparatory sensory information has been demonstrated to reduce anxieties in intensive care unit patients (Shi et al., 2003) and it is likely that such information will produce similar benefits in surgical patients (Carr, 2007).

Perceived loss of control

There is the potential for a series of events to occur from the point of admission that effectively threaten the individual's status and identity while absorbing them into the institution which can result in the individual's normal sense of autonomy and control being eliminated. For example, the patient has their clothes removed, wrist tabs applied and visitors restricted; this removes the individual's self-identity. According to Bonica (1990) this can result in some patients feeling that they have lost personal control over the situation, ensuring a sense of helplessness. Apart from anecdotal material the evidence for this is limited.

In threatening situations individuals adopt coping strategies in their desire for control over the situation

(Miller, 1987). Salmon (1994) divides coping strategies into patients who cope with a stressor by avoiding thinking about it ('avoiders') and those who confront the stressor by finding out what they can and using the information to think things through ('sensitizers'). Such differences help explain the diversity of decision-making among patients who report pain after surgery. For example, almost two-thirds of patients in one observational study (Manias et al., 2006) were passive in their pain management, which included pain assessment; and less than a fifth actually negotiated care.

Why assess acute pain?

If acute pain is to be expected and is part of a normal protective function, then why is it important to assess it? From a humanitarian perspective, failure to treat pain is ethically and morally unacceptable. Failure or inadequate pain assessment make a major contribution to the inadequacies associated with pain management. Other reasons for assessing pain include:

- determining the intensity, quality and duration of the pain;
- to aid diagnosis;
- to assist in determining the choice of analgesia;
- to evaluate the effectiveness of different therapies;
- to assist in the monitoring of clinical practice.

> ### Activity 4.3
>
>
>
> Think of a patient you have looked after with severe acute pain. What benefits could be derived from a formal assessment of that patient's pain?

Some of the issues you may have identified may correlate with a study that was carried out by Gould et al. (1992) in a large teaching hospital in Wales. They found that benefits of assessment included:

- preventing pain from building up, since pain can be treated while it is still moderate;
- provides evidence for the efficacy of the treatment given, enabling refinement of the patient's pain control;

- increases awareness to the patient's pain and displays interest in the patient's pain;
- reduces tendency to make assumptions when assessing pain;
- increases autonomy, enabling the patient to express their pain experience, which they may not feel able to do independently;
- increases the number of patients receiving analgesia therefore improving pain management and showing the patient that health care professionals believe in their reports of pain.

How often should acute pain be assessed?

The NHMRC (1998) suggest that patients' pain and response to treatment should be assessed at least every two hours for the first 24–48 hours following major surgery, and should be tailored to the patient's need in order to evaluate the efficacy of the analgesia. This therefore gives more specific guidelines for the frequency of pain assessment in nursing practice while allowing room for professional judgement and individualizing the regime for the patient.

> ### Activity 4.4
>
>
>
> Consider the organization you work in and answer the following questions. If you do not know the answers you may need to speak to someone with a designated interest in acute pain, such as a specialist nurse or an anaesthetist.
>
> - Is there a policy on the frequency of pain assessment in the area in which you work?
> - If so what is this?
> - How do you record pain assessment?
> - Is it formally recorded in the patient's notes or on a particular chart?
> - Are pain assessments audited?
> - If so how frequently?
> - What type of information is gathered?

In 2000 the Royal College of Anaesthetists produced an audit recipe book entitled *Raising the Standard*. The second edition of this information pack published in 2006 gives examples of various audits, best practice, suggested indicators, proposed standards and suggested data to be collected for various procedures within anaesthetics and critical care areas. These guidelines are a useful starting point when thinking of auditing pain management practices.

Some of the suggested indicators for acute pain management for the non-post-operative patient by the Royal College of Anaesthetists (2006: 242) include:

- *100% patients with acute pain should have a completed record of pain scores.*
- *< 10% patients should have an unacceptable peak or average pain score.*
- *Of patients with an unacceptable score, 100% should receive treatment within 15 min of the score being documented.*
- *> 95% patients requiring treatment should have a reduced pain score within 30 minutes of treatment. This should be documented on the chart.*
- *95% of staff should have received training within the past 12 months.*
- *100% of clinical areas should have current relevant guidelines for managing acute pain.*

As can be seen from the suggested indicators, pain assessment is an essential observation to be made by the health care professional if we are to seriously address the pain. How often, then, is dictated by the initial assessment of pain and the individual's response to management, and reassessment at times suggested within the indicators.

Key point

'Pain is the Fifth Vital Sign' is a widespread campaign that aims to encourage nurses to assess pain at the same time they record temperature, pulse, blood pressure and respiration.

When should pain be assessed?

There are four assessment times that are important (AHCPR, 1994):

1. Initially, to understand the pain and develop a plan of care.
2. At a suitable interval following an intervention, for example, 15–30 minutes after parenteral drug administration, one hour following oral drug administration, and immediately after a complementary treatment such as massage or acupuncture.
3. At regular intervals after treatment begins.
4. At a report of change in the description, location or intensity of the pain.

The assessment process can often be the start of helping the patient to manage their pain in a more effective manner. For example, in some cases of neuropathic pain and the majority of patients with back pain, giving explanations, where appropriate, that pain is not associated with progressive tissue damage can often begin to give the patient confidence to increase their activity and be more willing to take responsibility for the management of their pain.

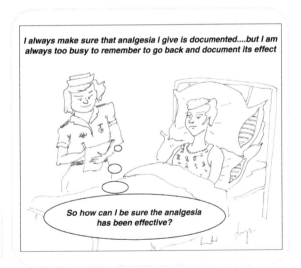

I always make sure that analgesia I give is documented....but I am always too busy to remember to go back and document its effect

So how can I be sure the analgesia has been effective?

How should acute pain be assessed?

Methods for nurses carrying out pain assessment need to be clear since according to the AHCPR (1992) recording patient responses to the question 'How is your pain?' invites misunderstandings. This question is ambiguous as it could generate hundreds of different responses from different patients, which is unhelpful in the acute setting when a valid and reliable response that can be recorded is required. Assessment of pain in such a non-structured way has been associated with pain underestimation (Lorenz et al., 2009). Even the manner or context in which a question is asked can be ambiguous or biased. For example, consider the two following questions asked by a nurse who has just come on duty.

'It's been four days since your operation Mr Smith, is your pain improving?'
'How much pain are you in Mr Smith?'

The former question could be perceived as loaded since it implies that since it is four days since his operation the pain should be improving whereas the latter question is automatically assuming that the patient is in pain.

Perhaps the following offers an alternative:

'Have you any pain when you are moving Mr Smith?'
'If so, is the pain mild, moderate or severe?'

These questions first assess whether or not the patient has pain on movement rather than rest which is a much more accurate assessment of pain since pain relief can be tailored to allow appropriate function. Effective analgesia is a prerequisite to good recovery as the problems associated with immobility are minimized. Assessing pain on movement is important where patients have to perform exercises for a smooth rehabilitation (Sloman et al., 2005).

If the patient has pain on movement then the pain can be described in exact terms using the words mild, moderate or severe. These words can then be charted or correlated with a numerical scale: 0 – no pain, 1 – mild pain, 2 – moderate pain and 3 – severe pain. It is essential that all staff consistently use the same tool on the same patient when assessing pain so improvements or otherwise in the patient's pain can be detected. It would be unhelpful to assess pain using a 0–3 scale, give analgesia for moderate pain then a colleague reassess the pain using a 0–10 scale because for this patient the assessment and subsequent evaluation of the treatment would not be consistent.

There are many pain assessment tools available to nurses. An acute pain assessment tool should be simple, valid and reliable (AHCPR, 1992) in order to reduce error and obtain information quickly. Validity

means that the tool accurately measures the intensity of pain while reliability means that the tool consistently measures pain intensity over time.

Pain assessment tools

Before using a pain assessment tool it is useful to consider the cause of the acute pain since this may reflect the choice of tool and the management required. In many cases the cause of the acute pain is obvious such as in the case of post-operative pain and trauma. However, in some cases such as acute abdominal pain or back pain, the cause of the pain may not be obvious and a diagnosis may not be certain. As we have already seen pain is influenced by the tissue that is injured so that different pains differ in their characteristics; for example, deep tissue damage produces a different pain experience to superficial damage and acute pain is different to chronic pain. These characteristics need to be considered when selecting an appropriate pain tool.

Additionally, depending on the type of pain, you may want a tool that offers a degree of individuality or is multidimensional; that is, assessing more than just severity. Tools should also be appropriate for a person's developmental, physical, emotional and cognitive cognition. In an acute setting a basic assessment of the location, intensity and influencing factors are usually required. It is important that the assessment tool should prompt the assessor to measure pain against functional ability; for example, movement, deep breathing or coughing rather than just scoring pain at rest.

Subjective measurements

Subjective measurements of the patient's description of pain are often the most reliable indicator of the presence and severity of pain. Factors such as the cause as mentioned previously, type of pain, duration, intensity, quality and influencing factors are important. In practice there are three types of tool that are used the most in assessing acute pain in the surgical setting. These are the *verbal rating scale (VRS)*, the *visual analogue scale (VAS)* and the *numerical rating scale (NRS)*.

Simple graded pain assessment charts are seen as being reliable and valid for use with patients therefore it makes sense to apply this tool to practice. See Fig. 4.3 for a sample pain assessment chart that could be included with the main observation chart along with other relevant assessment such as nausea and sedation.

Verbal rating scales

Communication plays an important role in assessing patients' post-operative pain when using an assessment chart. In Fig. 4.3, we have included a VRS that uses only four categories of pain severity from which to choose. In our example the adjectives mild, moderate and severe are given alongside a score for no pain. Other versions have more gradations on them, which allow for a fuller expression of the pain experience. In Jensen and Karoly (2001) a range of VRS are described: one is a four-point score similar to our version; another is also a four-point score but it uses more words to describe each category, from 'no pain at all' to 'pain that could not be more severe'; a third is a five-point score that splits severe pain into 'severe'

Pain assessment score

Ask the patient 'Which word best describes your pain on movement?' Put an X in the appropriate box below.

No pain	**0**
Mild pain	**1**
Moderate pain	**2**
Severe pain	**3**
Sleeping	**S**

Pain scale / chart:

Date	4/5/10	4/5/10	4/5/10	4/5/10	4/5/10	4/5/10	5/5/10	5/5/10	5/5/10	5/5/10
Time	10am	12md	4pm	6pm	7pm	10pm	2am	6am	10am	12md
If pain score is 2 or 3 then analgesia should be given										
3	X									
2		X	X							
1				X	X	X		X	X	X
0							S			

Figure 4.3 Example of a pain chart

and 'very severe'; while the fourth is a 15-point scale. This last scale moves through the spectrum of the pain experience through several very fine distinctions. For example, in the range from no pain to mild covered in our example, we have five grades: 'extremely weak', 'very weak' 'weak', 'very mild' and 'mild'. This is a very discriminating scale and has been used in both research and clinical practice but like all scales one has to consider two factors, practicality and accuracy. We would consider a four- or five-point scale to be more than practical in an acute pain setting where time is an issue in getting an assessment.

The VRS uses a **rank scoring** method and, such methods have been criticized as they assume equal weighting between the intervals (Jenson and Karoly, 2001). If you consider the difference between two points on our four-point scale described above, it becomes problematic when we try and quantify the difference between 'mild pain' and 'no pain' or between 'mild pain' and 'moderate pain'. This can cause problems when we want to monitor the effectiveness of a treatment, particularly around deciding how big an improvement we get. For example, if someone's pain decreases from severe to moderate pain, is that as big an effect as if their pain decreases from moderate to mild? A patient in moderate pain will, we imagine, still experience a large amount of distress and suffering even if they can function; whereas, someone in mild pain may be quite happy to tolerate this, rather than face the consequences of more treatment for their pain, such as side-effects from their medication.

Patients also often use other descriptors for their pain and this can be problematic when carers use their own interpretation of the patient's choice to translate the score onto the chart (Manias et al., 2006). The implication for practice is that patient education is an important consideration when using a pain assessment tool. Furthermore, health professionals must become skilled in using the pain assessment tool available to them, if accurate pain scores are to be obtained.

VAS

With a VAS, the patient is shown a 100 mm horizontal or vertical line. The end points are usually labelled 'no pain' or 'worst pain imaginable' (see Fig. 4.4). The patient is then asked to put a mark on the line to show how much pain they are in. The score is then calculated by measuring from the 'no pain' end of the line in centimetres or millimetres to where the patient has marked. This scale has become a recognized and validated research tool as it compares well with other methods of assessing pain, allows repeated records to be easily obtained, and shows great sensitivity to treatment effects (Jensen and Karoly, 2001). Some patients may not find this scale as easy to use as the verbal and numerical rating scales, and it is reported to be more time-consuming to use than a VRS (Cork et al., 2004). However, there are now several mechanical and electronic VAS devices commercially available that mean the patient just has to move a cursor for a reading to be obtained. These overcome many of these opportunities for error and delay. In its favour, a review of the literature by Coll et al. (2004) advocates the VAS as the best tool for surgical pain assessment because the:

> VAS was found to be methodologically sound, conceptually simple, easy to administer and unobtrusive to the respondent. On these grounds, the VAS seems to be most suitable for measuring intensity of pain after day surgery.
>
> (Coll et al., 2004: 124)

The VAS is used widely in research studies into pain and other symptoms. You can for example change the descriptors at either end to nausea and measure this in the same way as pain. Sometimes the scale is broken down to 11 divisions in a numerical rating scale (Fig. 4.5) but this does not have the same amount of sensitivity to change as seen in the VAS.

NRS

Like the VRS and the VAS the numerical rating scale is validated for both research and clinical practice. It also seems to be very acceptable to patients and its use is widespread as it is easy to explain and to administer. It does not require the patient to mark a piece of paper or manipulate a device like the VAS (Jensen and Karoly, 2001). Instead, people are asked to score the intensity of their pain on a 0 to 10 scale with the understanding that 0 represents no pain, and 10 the worst pain ever. It is relatively simple to use and

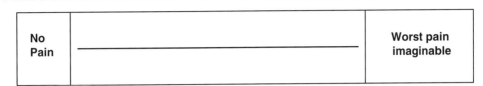

Figure 4.4 Visual analogue scale

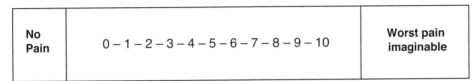

Figure 4.5 Numerical graphic rating scale

has accuracy across a wide range of patients, including children (von Baeyer et al., 2009) and pain situations. For this reason Jensen and Karoly (2001) advocate its widespread use, although it does not provide the same degree of sensitivity to changes in pain intensity as the VAS. In our experiences we have also come across situations where, despite careful explanation, patients mix up the end points.

Effectiveness of pain assessment

The effect of implementing a pain assessment was studied by Gould et al. (1992). They found that after the introduction of pain assessment and an hourly algorithm for the administration of intramuscular opioid, fewer patients received no analgesia and the average dose of intramuscular analgesia increased in the first 24 hours post-op. This suggests more patients had their pain assessed and patients' reports of pain were acted on.

These findings are supported by Harmer and Davies (1998) who carried out a study based on the work by Gould et al. (1992). They found a significant decrease in pain at rest and on movement after a formal assessment tool was introduced along with an algorithm for intermittent intramuscular opioid analgesia and staff education. The overall implication from this study was that patients received better analgesia and had greater satisfaction with their

management when pain was assessed using an assessment tool. There is also evidence that introducing simple pain assessment tools, such as the VAS, increases the frequency of pain diagnoses when compared to just asking people 'Do you have pain?' (Hosam et al., 2001).

Pain assessment in children

As with pain assessment and management in adults, there are many misconceptions regarding pain in children such as:

- infants do not feel pain;
- children tolerate pain better than adults;
- children cannot tell you where it hurts;
- behavioural manifestations of pain reflect the pain intensity;
- opioids are dangerous for children.

It can be difficult to assess children's pain adequately because of their limited ability to express their pain particularly in very young children and neonates. However, just as with adults the rights of children and their families must be respected and this includes enabling them to participate in pain assessment as part of involving them in their own pain management. To achieve this it is important to learn and use the language of children if you want them to be able to self-report their pain. Where they are unable to communicate then attention to behavioural cues in pre-verbal children and children with developmental problems is important. Such methods should be appropriate to the cognitive development of the child in order to facilitate their expression of pain. The cause of the pain should also be taken into account as the pathology may give clues as to the expected intensity and type of pain and hence its treatment.

Involving the family as partners in the care is also important. Parents should be actively involved in assessment as they are familiar with their child's normal behaviour and language and can provide accurate judgements on their condition which can promote early recognition and accurate assessment of pain. For example, the words children use to describe their pain vary and a parent or carer can help identify those their child usually uses. Where parents and children are involved then pain management improves as does their satisfaction with pain management (Wilson and Doyle, 1996; Franck et al., 2007)

A variety of pain assessment strategies such as questioning, evaluating behaviour, and using an appropriate pain rating scale, such as a NRS (Jensen and Karoly, 2001) or the Wong-Baker FACES pain rating scale (Fig. 4.6) are needed (Hockenberry and Wilson, 2009).

The FACES scale consists of six cartoon faces ranging from smiling for 'no pain' to crying for 'worst pain'. It is important with this scale that it is explained to the child that the faces relate to someone who feels happy because there is no pain (hurt) or sad because there is some or a lot of pain. The FACES scale has been successfully used for children from the age of 3 upwards. It has also been widely adapted and used in other groups of patients. However, it does require a certain developmental level to have been reached and is therefore unsuitable for very young children such as toddlers and babies.

In those who are unable to help with an assessment of their pain, it is not possible to use self-report as a measurement of pain. There are a number of ways around this. Facial expressions of pain may be utilized (Carr and Mann, 2000) but this approach does have limitations and does require close observation and education of staff. Other alternatives include objective rating scales. These include the modified objective pain score (MOPS) which is designed to be used in children from birth to the age of 4 who are non-verbal, but has been used in up to 12-year-olds (Wilson and Doyle, 1996). It includes five criteria: crying, movement, agitation, posture and verbal expression. In some versions the verbal criterion is replaced by facial expression (smiling to grimacing). While there might be other reasons for these behavioural changes, we feel that it is entirely reasonable to assume that the reason for this change occurring during a procedure or after an operation is down to pain, especially if the child is unable to communicate.

Wong-Baker Faces Pain Rating Scale

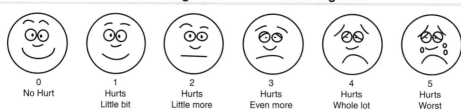

Brief word instructions: Point to each face using the words to describe the pain intensity. Ask the child to choose face that best describes own pain and record the appropriate number.

Original instructions: Explain to the person that each face is for a person who feels happy because he has no pain (hurt) or sad because he has some or a lot of pain. Face 0 is very happy because he doesn't hurt at all. Face 1 hurts just a little bit. Face 2 hurts a little more. Face 3 hurts even more. Face 4 hurts a whole lot. Face 5 hurts as much as you can imagine, although you don't have to be crying to feel this bad. Ask the person to choose the face that best describes how he is feeling. Rating scale is recommended for persons age 3 years and older.

Figure 4.6 Wong Baker FACES pain rating scale
Source: Hockenberry, M.J. and Wilson, D. (2009) *Wong's Essentials of Pediatric Nursing*, 8th edn. St. Louis, MI: Mosby. Reprinted with permission. @ Mosby.

Activity 4.5

Select two of the pain assessment tools described so far in this chapter. Try using them when assessing 10 patients in your clinical practice. If a pain assessment tool is in use in your clinical area use that as one of the two tools. Compare your chosen pain assessment tools by asking yourself the following questions.

- How easy are they to use?
- Do they encourage the patient or client or family to be involved in the pain assessment process?
- Are there any other advantages and disadvantages to each tool?

Criteria	Advantages	Disadvantages
Age	No barrier	Barrier
Time	Brief	Too time-consuming
Detail	Comprehensive	Limited
Ease of use	Easy to understand	Ambiguous
Staff preparation	No or little preparation needed	Staff education required to ensure reliability in use

Table 4.1 Criteria for evaluating pain assessment tools

To be successful a pain assessment tool should be easy to use. Some of the aspects that need to be considered in order to ensure this include (Jacox et al., 1994):

- simplicity;
- clarity;
- proven reliability and validity.

A tool that meets these criteria should be easy for both members of the multidisciplinary team and patients to use. It is also more likely to be successfully used.

Additional considerations might be the introduction of cultural bias. A tool must be appropriate for clients from different national and ethnic groups, and where necessary, available in several languages. Some scales are more easily adapted than others. Numeric and visual analogue scales can be appropriate in any cultural setting and are easy to use if explained carefully. However, word-based scales or facial scales, particularly ones that use photographs, may be more difficult and will require more care when using them among people with different skin colour or ethnicity or where language barriers exist.

Reflect again on your use of the two tools and consider how each met the criteria in Table 4.1.

When assessing acute pain remember the six golden rules of acute pain assessment (Table 4.2)!

1. Always *assess* pain
2. Always *ask* the patient
3. *All* people should always use the *same* pain assessment tool on the *same* patient
4. Always assess pain on *movement* or *deep breathing* or *coughing* and not just at *rest*
5. Always *document* the patient's pain assessment
6. Always *evaluate* the intervention using the *same* pain assessment tool

Table 4.2 The golden rules of pain assessment

The assessment of chronic pain

Having explored the principles of assessing acute pain, we now examine chronic pain. Before proceeding complete the following activity which encourages you to clarify the differences between these two types of pain.

Activity 4.6

Using your experience make a short list of some of the things you feel differentiates acute and chronic pain.

> **Case study 4.1**
>
> Two patients undergoing an exploratory laparotomy for 'a growth'
>
> The excision is exactly the same and one would anticipate that the visceral damage and manipulation of tissue be similar. One patient has an inoperable carcinoma and the second has a benign condition.
>
> Post-operatively both patients suffer pain but it is suggested that the significance of pain in the two patients is somewhat different.
>
> After the operation both patients are informed of their diagnosis and prognosis.

Your answer may have included some of the following (see Table 4.3):

Acute	Chronic
Recent onset	Pain which has lasted for long periods, generally more than six months, or persisting beyond the normal injury healing process
Causal relationship between injury and disease	May not always be an identifiable cause for the pain
Possible to estimate duration	Duration of chronic pain unlimited – no idea of the time scale involved.

Table 4.3 Differences between acute and chronic pain

From your answers you will see that the focus of pain assessment may differ for each of the groups, based on the time scale and psychosocial factors involved.

At first sight one may well consider that in acute pain, the prevalence of sensory factors will take precedence over the emotive response, whereas in chronic pain states, where one would anticipate that the persistence of pain generally outlives the effects of any organic damage, it would be reasonable to assume that the behavioural factors and the patient's reaction to the painful condition would be more relevant. It is certainly the case that it is extremely uncommon for chronic pain to exist in the absence of behavioural

changes, but equally so it appears that the perception of acute pain is influenced by factors other than the actual nociceptive experience.

It may be helpful to consider the acute pain scenario in Case study 4.1 to focus on the 'meaning' of pain and the effect this has on an individual.

For the patient who has been told that his laparotomy has revealed a benign condition, the pain signifies damage due to surgery which will be short lived and will go with time and he will 'live to fight another day'. The other patient who has been told that he has a cancer that cannot be removed may well perceive the pain experience as being possibly never-ending and associated with his ultimate death. It appears that the actual amount of pain experienced even in an acute pain situation is not purely related to the actual surgery performed, but the emotive factors also have a role to play.

If we accept that the assessment of pain should encompass several aspects of an individual's pain experience, then it is necessary to read a balance between assessing the sensory aspect of pain and the emotive aspects. Current practice within the UK is that the emotive aspects of acute pain are not routinely measured, but alterations in the severity of pain are measured with the aid of simple pain scales as discussed earlier in this chapter. In the past attempts have been made to introduce complex pain assessment tools but these have proved to be too unwieldy for regular use on busy clinical areas. This is in contrast to the assessment of chronic pain whereby reliance on simple sensory assessment tools without considering behavioural and psychosocial factors are generally considered to produce an incomplete assessment.

The process of assessment in chronic nonmalignant pain

Whatever the cause, the effect of chronic pain on the patient tends to be more pervasive than that of acute pain. It profoundly affects the patient's mood, personality and social relationships. People with chronic pain typically experience depression, sleep disturbance, fatigue and decreased overall physical functioning. As a result pain is only one of many issues that must be addressed in the assessment of patients with chronic pain (Ashburn and Staats, 1999), hence the assessment should cover several areas.

In other words, reconsidering the International Association for the Study of Pain (IASP) definition of pain (Chapter 1), the assessment of chronic painful conditions must look at the sensory aspect of the pain, the patient's emotional condition and their reaction to the pain.

In assessing the patient experiencing chronic pain, it is often helpful to utilize a multidisciplinary assessment, which will include medical, physiotherapy and psychological input. Many pain clinics will use questionnaires, which are delivered to the patient before their assessment, and these questionnaires often include screening tools to assess the effect of pain on mood, function and quality of life.

Some aspects that chronic pain questionnaires focus on are as follows.

The character of pain

Location

Pain may arise in a particular location because of an underlying problem in the immediate area, or, some pains can be 'referred' and felt in another part of the body. In patients with low back pain and sciatica, pain may be felt as a dull ache in the lower spine, but may also be felt as a burning sensation along the outside of the leg. Pain may also be presenting from a multitude of sources and it is not unusual to have several painful areas at the same time (Davies et al., 1998). It is important to let the person know that this is not uncommon, and let them locate their pain on a body chart, such as the long form of the Wisconsin Brief Pain Inventory (BPI) (Daut et al., 1983).

Description

Pain can be experienced and described in a number of ways: a dull ache, throbbing, tenderness, stabbing, burning. Each description gives significant clues as to the possible cause of the pain. For example, burning often relates to nerve pain, such as that seen in sciatica. It is important that the person in pain describes what it feels like as exactly as possible (Melzack, 1987), although there can be problems obtaining this information. The McGill Pain Questionnaire (MPQ) was specifically developed to generate this type of detail although there appear to be differences between genders in the number of descriptors chosen, with women choosing more than men (Strong et al., 2009).

Time-related factors

Questions such as 'How long have you had the pain?', 'When did it begin?' and 'When is it better or worse?' can give diagnostic clues that will assist in planning treatment.

Intensity

The level of pain and its intensity must be assessed and as mentioned in the earlier section to this chapter, there are a range of scales that can be useful when making this assessment. That discussion is equally applicable to the measure of intensity in chronic pain and so will not be repeated here.

Influencing factors

This involves asking the questions 'What makes the pain better?' or 'What makes the pain worse?' Again, these factors can give diagnostic clues but also, more importantly, may suggest some non-pharmacological methods of easing the pain. In the case of chronic pain the person may have had their pain for a long time and may have tried many forms of treatment. It is important to find out what they have tried in the past and what has or has not worked for them (Dunn, 2000).

Psychosocial assessment

The factors to which people attribute their pain will influence their response to it and the patient's adaptation to their pain will have a major influence on its character (Blyth et al., 2007). In terms of chronic pain, it is important to remember that usually the pain will not be eradicated only controlled, so the person's understanding of their pain will have a great influence on their long-term management. Acknowledging the contribution of psychosocial factors in the development and maintenance of chronic pain is the key to helping patients. In order to do this assessment strategies that encompass social, family and work history, as well as beliefs and attitudes to pain and an assessment of behaviours, are needed. For example, you may wish to measure the impact of pain on the patient and their family and also the extent to which the family reinforces pain behaviours that add to the problem. In chronic pain it is also useful to establish the extent of fear avoidance behaviour that is displayed (Grotle et al., 2004) and to ascertain whether or not they feel that the pain they experience is a reflection of ongoing disease.

Functional assessment

A functional assessment generally looks at how the person's pain disables someone by interfering with activities of daily living including mobility, sleeping, eating and working and leisure activities. The long form of the Wisconsin Brief Pain Inventory (Daut et al, 1983) and the newer short form (Cleeland, 1989) lists the various functional aspects that may be affected by pain and quantifies the degree of interference, providing a comprehensive, consistent and efficient way of structuring an assessment. If an area is affected, one should explore further to define how specifically the pain interferes with the activity. For example, if sleeping is affected, questions such as 'Is there difficulty getting to sleep or staying asleep?' should be asked. Obtaining information about the degree of difficulty, especially if the interference can be quantified, allows evaluation of the care plan at an objective level. Defining the specific manner of interference; for example, falling asleep but not being able to sleep through the night, may provide goals to work towards in the pain management plan (Dunn, 2000).

Recently, the emphasis on functional assessment has shifted from what someone cannot do to what someone in chronic pain can do (Verbunt et al., 2009). This is a move away from disability assessment to

competence evaluation. Verbunt et al. (2009) extensively reviewed several established functional assessment tools to see if they reflected this change in attitude and came to the conclusion that most focused on disability and adaptation to disability rather than on the 'daily activity level' of people in pain. Only those tools that measured physical movement met their criteria for assessment of activity and they identified a need to develop tools that evaluate other aspects of function rather than just the physical.

> **Key point**
>
> Many chronic pain tools focus on what people are unable to do. Perhaps a better way would be to focus on what they can do.

Pain history assessment

These tools look at the patient's perception of their pain, what methods of pain management have been tried, and what has been successful. From this aspect of questioning, the patient's frustration and anger can become apparent from the words and terms used. Patients often say, 'Nothing's been done! Nobody cares'.

In reality the patient may have been fully investigated by many specialists, but no definitive cause for the pain identified. This frustration and anger is commonly seen in the pain clinics to which patients are often referred when no other management strategies have been found. Taking a complete pain history can often save time by avoiding duplication of treatment methods.

Questionnaire methods

A number of pain assessment questionnaires have been developed; here we compare four.

(1) McGill Pain Questionnaire (MPQ)
Melzack and Torgerson (1971) developed the MPQ. Descriptive words were classified into three classes and 20 sub-classes:

- sensory qualities of the pain; for example, aching, stabbing, sharp

- affective qualities of the pain; for example, tiring, cruel
- evaluative qualities of the pain describing the subjective intensity; for example, unbearable

Patients are asked to select one word from each sub-class to describe their pain. Within each sub-class words are arranged in order of increasing pain; for example, hot, burning, scalding, and searing.

Measurements derived include:

- Pain rating index (PRI) – a scoring system in which differing values are given to words in a group and a total score is obtained. This indicates whether the pain is purely nociceptive or has neuropathic elements.
- Number of words chosen (NWC) indicates the burden of the pain.
- Present pain index (PPI) – an indicator of overall pain intensity at the time of examination. Using a numerical rating score (0 equals no pain whereas 5 equals excruciating pain).

The MPQ provides a statistically significant assessment tool for assessing painful conditions. Its main disadvantage is the length of the questionnaire and the time taken to complete it. In our experience it takes at least 30 minutes to administer this questionnaire to a fully cognizant adult and this limits its applicability in clinical practice. Since its introduction the MPQ has been used extensively and experience suggests that it provides precise information on the sensory, affective and evaluative aspects of pain experience as well as being able to discriminate between different pain problems (Melzack, 1975). Researchers from various countries have translated it, tested its reliability and validity and have found it to be a valuable and sensitive tool. It is still viewed as a gold standard in pain assessment.

② Short form McGill Pain questionnaire
A shortened form of the MPQ (SF-MPQ) has also been developed (Melzack, 1987) for use in the clinical and research situations which require a more rapid acquisition of data than the standard MPQ. It consists of 15 words, 11 from the sensory and 4 from the affective sub-classes. PPI and visual analogues scales are also included to assess the overall pain intensity. The SF-MPQ has been demonstrated to be as valid as the long form of the MPQ (LF-MPQ) although it is most reliable for intensity and sensory discriminative (Wright et al., 2001).

③ Short form 36 health survey (SF-36)
This questionnaire includes an assessment of mood, function and quality of life. This aims at finding out what is bothering the patient about their pain and the impact the pain has on their day-to-day activities. This is particularly useful to do in chronic pain as it allows us to compare their specific perceptions as to the cause of their pain and its meaning to them with their general perceptions on health.

Attention should also be paid to the patient's interpretations of previous medical explanations about their condition. For example, a description of degenerative disc disease may imply to the patient that their back condition will inevitably worsen and consequently they should avoid activities that reproduce their pain.

SF-36 has been used widely in research into the characteristics of chronic pain sufferers and more recently to measure outcomes of interventions such as pain management programmes. The SF-36 bodily pain dimension is viewed as being less reliable than a single intensity score such as a VAS or NRS (Jensen, 2003). However, it is a multidimensional pain score not just an intensity score so this is an unfair comparison and it also has advantages of a huge database supporting it allowing cross-comparisons between patients and populations, a factor that intensity scores do not allow.

④ The short form brief pain inventory (BPI)
This is another quickly completed scoring system, taking less than 5 minutes to complete. It scores worst, average and current pain intensity on numerical rating scales, medication usage and efficacy, and quantifies the impact on quality of life. It was originally developed for use in

	McGill Pain Questionnaire (standard and short form)	**SF 36**	**Brief pain inventory**
Purpose	Pain generic instrument	To assess quality of life measures for generic health problems	To assess the severity of pain and the impact of pain on daily functions
Population	All except children and neonates	Adult and adolescent (age 14 and older)	Adults with cancer pain and pain due to other chronic diseases
Assessment areas	Sensory, affective and other qualitative components of current pain	Quality of life. Impact of health problems on daily function (both physical and emotional), bodily pain, general health perception, vitality, social functioning, mental health. Over the last four weeks (standard version) or the last week (acute version)	Severity of pain, impact of pain on daily function, location of pain, pain medications, and amount of pain relief in the past 24 hours or the past week
Responsiveness	To changes in pain produced by different interventions	The health benefits produced by different interventions	Behavioural and pharmacological pain interventions
Method	Usually interviewer-administered as it is necessary to maintain consistency of the procedure. Some complex items and terms. MPQ: pain rating scale with 102 words sorted into three classes. The short form has 15 words	Self-administered or interviewer-administered (by a trained interviewer in person or by telephone). Also via computer program. 36 items.	Self-report, interview, or via an interactive Voice Response System (IVR) Long form 51 items; Short form 15 items.
Time required	MPQ 20–30 minutes; short form 5–10 minutes	5–10 minutes	Five minutes (short form), 10 minutes (long form)

Scoring	Several scoring methods. Most commonly used involves summing scale weights for the words chosen	Algorithmic scores on eight domains of health and summary scores for physical and mental health as well as a general health index	No scoring algorithm, but 'worst pain' or the arithmetic mean of the four severity items is used as a measure of pain severity and the arithmetic mean of the seven interference items is used as a measure of pain interference
Validation	Is widely regarded as the 'gold standard' for pain questionnaires. The MPQ has been extensively translated	SF-36 has been validated in over 50 different countries and in seven different age groups	Has been validated in 12 different languages by examining the consistency of its two factor structure (factors: severity of pain and impact of pain).

Table 4.4 Comparison of four questionnaires

oncology and arthritis patients, but has since been used in numerous chronic nonmalignant conditions (University of Texas MD Anderson Cancer Center, 2009).

This provides a concise way to communicate information to the variety of people involved in addressing the person's pain. While giving a 'snapshot' in time about the person and their pain, the form also provides a baseline by which the effectiveness of a pain management plan can be judged.

Pain diaries and journals

Some patients find it helpful to complete a pain diary. This is directed at charting the pain intensity using a numerical rating scale, recording activities of daily living and medications. These need to be filled in at the time to avoid distortion, but provide an estimate of how the patient functions in their normal environment. The use of a pain diary varies between patients and may become less reliable with time because of compliance. Another disadvantage is that it focuses the patient's attention more on the pain, and the limitations on life that the pain imposes. It also requires a level of literacy, comprehension and accuracy of

record-keeping, so may be unsuitable for some patients. There are no validated pain diaries or journals as these are by their nature individual and comparison across patients and groups is therefore not possible.

Chronic pain assessment in children

Chronic pain assessment in children is complicated by the age and development of the child and their interaction with the parents in much the same way as in acute and palliative pain. Furthermore, the way in which children perceive the cause and effect of pain changes as they mature. For example, a 5-year-old will describe a painful event in a different manner to a 12-year-old (Perquin et al., 2000).

In infants with no verbal skills this can be difficult, with the assessor relying on such gross measures as crying or motor withdrawal. These are measures of general distress, so are non-specific at best. Toddlers begin to develop localizing and other signs that are more indicative of pain, such as rubbing, as well as more complex although less specific behaviours such as lip smacking, and aggressive behaviours. From the age of 3 children begin to be able to cope with simple rating measures such as the FACES scale and colour matching. From about 5 years of age children can complete visual analogue and other simple scales. Multidimensional scales such as the MPQ have been validated for patients older than 12 (Dolin, 1996).

Children are likely to be exposed to the same types and syndromes of chronic pain as adults, although the extent may vary (Rowbotham, 2000). For example, chronic pains associated with ageing, such as osteoarthritis, will be lower. Common chronic pain problems in children include headaches. Migraines form a large subcategory of headaches and may also manifest as other chronic pain such as abdominal pain. Chronic pain in children can also be experienced as the result of trauma or injury (Chalkiadis, 2001) due to one of the arthropathies such as rheumatoid arthritis or as a result of a chronic condition such as Sickle Cell Disease. However, there is very little that is known about the incidence of chronic pain in this population.

Summary

This chapter has explored the nature of acute and chronic pain assessment. In particular we have looked at what makes chronic pain assessment different from acute pain assessment and consider, briefly, the difference between the assessment of adults and children. Emphasis has been placed on the benefits of making an assessment and making informed choices in terms of the assessment tool.

In chronic pain we cannot emphasize enough the importance of a detailed assessment that goes beyond simply measuring intensity. No one chronic pain assessment method is superior in all circumstances; nevertheless, a holistic assessment increases the likelihood that the pain will be understood and defined accurately and, most importantly, effectively addressed.

From the points we have discussed, you should now be able to:

- demonstrate an awareness of the benefits of acute pain assessment for the care of the person in acute pain;
- appreciate how an understanding of these benefits can contribute to the avoidance of health problems and complications in people with acute pain, particularly after surgery;
- evaluate different methods of assessing acute pain;
- demonstrate an understanding of the physical, psychological and sociological effects of chronic pain;
- appreciate how an understanding of these elements is vital in order to undertake holistic, effective pain assessment in chronic nonmalignant pain;
- identify different methods of assessing chronic pain.

Reflective activity

As a conclusion to this chapter consider how knowledge of this theory will help you in your future practice. Try to be specific and use the following points/questions as a guide.

- *State* which elements of the chapter will help you in your future practice.
- *Elaborate:* be specific in terms of how this knowledge and understanding can be used in practice.
- *Give examples:* of care events which would benefit from what you have learnt.
- What are the *implications* if you change the way you practise?

You may prefer to use a reflective model such as Gibbs's (1988) to guide your reflection (see Appendix at the end of this book). Think of a specific example as the starting point. Describe the event and then proceed through the cycle. When analysing the situation draw on this chapter's theory to support your discussion and demonstrate your understanding. As a result your reflection will examine the utilization and effectiveness of pain assessment.

References

Agency for Health Care Policy and Research (AHCPR) (1992) *Acute Pain Management: Operative or Medical Procedures and Trauma.* Rockville MD: AHCPR No. 92-0032.

Agency for Health Care Policy and Research (1994) *Management of Cancer Pain.* Rockville, MD: AHCPR No. 94-0592.

Allcock, N. (1996) Factors effecting the assessment of postoperative pain: a literature review, *Journal of Advanced Nursing*, 24:6: 1144–51.

Ashburn, M.A. and Staats, P.S. (1999) Management of chronic pain, *The Lancet*, 353: 9167, 1865–9.

Audit Commission (1997) *National Report. Anaesthesia under Examination: The Efficiency and Effectiveness of Anaesthesia and Pain Relief Services in England and Wales.* London: Belmont Press.

Baylock, H.T. (1968) Psychological and cultural influences on the reaction to pain, *Nurse Forum*, 7: 271–72.

Blyth, F.M., Macfarlane, G.J. and Nicholas, M.K. (2007) The contribution of psychosocial factors to the development of chronic pain: the key to better outcomes for patients? *Pain*, 129(1–2): 8–11.

Bonica J. (1990) Definition and taxonomy of pain, in J. Bonica (ed.) *The Management of Pain*, 2nd edn Philadelphia, PA: Lea & Febiger.

Brockopp, D.Y., Downey, E., Powers, P., Vanderveer, B., Warden, S., Ryan, P. & Saleh, U. (2004) Nurses' clinical decision-making regarding the management of pain, *International Journal of Nursing Studies*, 41(6): 631–6.

Brunier, G., Carson, G. and Harrison, D.E. (1995) What do nurses know and believe about patients with pain? Results of a hospital survey, *Journal of Pain and Symptom Management*, 10(6): 436–45.

Carr, E. (2007) Barriers to effective pain management, *Journal of Perioperative Practice*, 17(5): 200.

Carr, E.C.J. and Mann, E.M. (2000) *Pain: Creative Approaches to Effective Management.* Basingstoke: Palgrave Macmillan.

Chalkiadis, G.A. (2001) Management of chronic pain in children, *Medical Journal of Australia*, 175: 476–9. Available online at www.mja.com.au/public/issues/175_09_051101/chalkiadis/chalkiadis.html. (accessed 1 July 2009).

Chernow, B. (1987) Hormonal responses to a graded surgical stress, *Archives of Internal Medicine*, 147: 1273–8.

Clarke, E.B, French, B, Bilodeau, M.L, Capasso, V.C, Edwards, A. and Empoliti, J. (1996) Pain management knowledge, attitudes and clinical practice: the impact of nurses, characteristics and education, *Journal of Pain and Symptom Management*, 11(1): 18–31.

Cleeland, C.S. (1989) Measurement of pain by subjective report, in C.R., Chapman and J.D. Loeser (eds) *Advances in Pain Research and Therapy*, pp. 391–403. 12: Issues in pain measurement. New York: Raven Press.

Clinical Standards Advisory Group (CSAG) (2000) *Services for Patients with Pain.* London: Clinical Standards Advisory Group, Her Majesty's Stationery Office (HMSO).

Closs, J., Briggs, M. and Everitt, V. (1997) Night-time pain, sleep and anxiety in postoperative orthopaedic patients, *Journal of Orthopaedic Nursing*, 1(2): 59–66.

Coll, A.-M., Ameen, J. and Mead, D. (2004) Postoperative pain assessment tools in day surgery: a critical review, *Journal of Advanced Nursing*, 46(2): 124–33.

Cork, R.C., Isaac, I., Elsharydah, A., Saleemi, S., Zavisca, F. and Alexander, L. (2004) A comparison of the verbal rating scale and the visual analog scale for pain assessment, *The Internet Journal of Anesthesiology*, 8(1).

Daut, R.L., Cleeland, C.S. and Flanery, R.C. (1983) The development of the Wisconsin Brief Pain Questionnaire to assess pain in cancer and other diseases, *Pain*, 17: 197–210.

Davies, H.T.O., Crombie, I.K. and Macrae, W.A. (1998) Where does it hurt? Describing the body locations of chronic pain, *European Journal of Pain*, 2(1): 69–80.

Defrin, R., Lotan, M. and Pick, C.G. (2006) The evaluation of acute pain in individuals with cognitive impairment: a differential effect of the level of impairment, *Pain*, 124(3): 312–20.

Dolin, S.J. (1996) The pain patient, in S.J. Dolin, N. Padfield and J. Paterman (eds) *Pain Clinic Manual* (p. 15). Oxford: Reed Educational and Professional Publishing.

Dunn V. (2000) The holistic assessment of the patient in pain, *Professional Nurse*, 15(12): 791–3.

Fordham, M.A. and Dunn, V. (1994) *Alongside the Person in Pain.* London: Bailliere Tindall.

Franck, L.S., Allen, A. and Oulton, K. (2007) Making pain assessment more accessible to children and parents: can greater involvement improve the quality of care? *The Clinical Journal of Pain*, 23(4): 331–8.

Giannoudis, P.V., Dinopoulos, H., Chalidis, B. and Hall, G.M. (2006) Surgical stress response, *Injury*, 37(5): pp. 3–9.

Gibbs, G. (1988) *Learning by Doing: A Guide to Teaching and Learning Methods.* Oxford: Further Education Unit. Oxford Polytechnic.

Gould, T.H., Crosby, D.L., Harmer, M, Lloyd, S.M., Lunn, J.N, Rees, G.A.D, Roberts, D.E. and Webster, J.A. (1992) Policy for controlling pain after surgery: effect of sequential changes in management, *British Medical Journal*, 305: 1187–93.

Grotle, M., Vøllestad, N.K., Veierød, M.B. and Brox, J.I. (2004) Fear-avoidance beliefs and distress in relation to disability in acute and chronic low back pain, *Pain*, 112(3): 343–52.

Hamers, J.P.H., Huijer Abu-Saad, H. Halfens, R.J.G. Schumacher JMN, (1994) Factors influencing nurses' pain assessment and interventions in children, *Journal of Advanced Nursing*, 20:5: 787–982.

Harmer, M, and Davies, K.A. (1998) The effect of education, assessment and a standardised prescription on postoperative pain management, *Anaesthesia*, 53: 424–30.

Hirsh, A. and Jensen, M. (2009) Nurses' self-awareness of their decision-making process for pain assessment and treatment, *The Journal of Pain*, 10(4, Supplement 1): S72.

Hockenberry, M.J. and Wilson, D. (2009) *Wong's Essentials of Pediatric Nursing*, 8th edn. St. Louis, MI: Mosby.

Hosam, K.K., Mohsen, P., Behnam, M., Philip, G. and John, E.M. (2001) Utilizing pain assessment scales increases the frequency of diagnosing pain among elderly nursing home residents, *Journal of Pain and Symptom Management*, 21(6): 450–5.

Hunter, S. (2000) Determination of moral negligence in the context of the undermedication of pain by nurses, *Nursing Ethics*, 7(5): 379–91.

Jacox, A., Carr, D.B. and Payne, R. et al. (1994) *Management of Cancer Pain, Clinical Practice Guideline No. 9*. Rockville, MD AHCPR No. 94-0592.

Jensen, M.P. (2003) The validity and reliability of pain measures in adults with cancer, *The Journal of Pain*, 4(1): 2–21.

Jensen, M.P. and Karoly, P. (2001) Self-report scales and procedures for assessing pain in adults, in D.C. Turk and R. Melzack (eds) *The Handbook of Pain Assessment* (pp. 15–34). New York: Guilford Press.

Lorenz, K.A., Sherbourne, C.D., Shugarman, L.R., Rubenstein, L.V., Wen, L., Cohen, A., Goebel, J.R., Hagenmeier, E., Simon, B., Lanto, A. and Asch, S.M. (2009) How reliable is pain as the fifth vital sign? *Journal of the American Board of Family Medicine*, 22(3), 291–8.

Manias, E., Botti, M. and Bucknall, T. (2006) Patients' decision-making strategies for managing postoperative pain, *The Journal of Pain*, 7(6): 428–37.

McQuay, H. and Moore, A. (1998) Acute Pain: Conclusion, in H. McQuay and A. Moore (eds) (1998) *An Evidence Based Resource For Pain Relief*. Oxford: Oxford University Press.

Melzack, R. (1975) The McGill Pain Questionnaire: major properties and scoring methods, *Pain*, 1: 277–99.

Melzack, R. (1987) The short form McGill Pain Questionnaire, *Pain*, 30: 191–97.

Melzack, R. and Torgerson, W.S. (1971) On the language of pain, *Anaesthesiology*, 34: 50–9.

Melzack, R. and Wall, P.D. (1965) Pain mechanisms: a new theory, *Science*, 150: 971–9.

Miller, S.M. (1987) Monitoring and blunting: validation of a questionnaire to assess styles of information seeking under threat, *Journal of Personality and Social Psychology*, 52: 345–53.

National Health and Medical Research Council (1998) *Acute Pain Management: Scientific Evidence*. Canberra: NHMRC.

Notcutt, W.G. (1997) What makes acute pain chronic? *Current Anaesthesia and Critical Care*, 8(2): 55–61.

Perquin, C.W., Hazebroek-Kampschreur, A.A.J.M., Hunfield, J.A.M., Bohnen, A.M., Van Suijlekom-Smit, L.W.A., Passchier, J. and van der Wouden, J.C. (2000) Pain in children and adolescents: a common experience, *Pain*, 87(1): 51–8.

Powell, A.E., Davies, H.T.O., Bannister, J. and Macrae, W.A. (2009) Challenge of improving postoperative pain management: case studies of three acute pain services in the UK National Health Service, *British Journal of Anaesthesia*, 102(6): 824–31.

Regnard, C.F.B. and Tempest, S. (1998) *A Guide to Symptom Relief in Advanced Disease*, 4th edn. Altrincham: Hochland and Hochland.

Rowbotham D.J. (2000) *Chronic Pain*. London: Martin Dunitz Ltd.

Royal College of Anaesthetists (2006) *Raising the Standard: A Compendium of Audit Recipes 2nd edn*. Available online at www.rcoa.ac.uk/index.asp?PageID=125&SearchStr=Raising%20the%20Standard (accessed 26 March 2010).

Royal College of Surgeons of England and College of Anaesthetists (1990) *Report of the Working Party on Pain after Surgery*, London.

Salmon, P. (1994) Psychological factors in surgical recovery, in H.B. Gibson (ed.) *Psychology, Pain and Anaesthesia*. London: Chapman & Hall.

Schafheutle, E.I. Cantrill, J.A. and Noyce, P.R. (2001) Why is pain management suboptimal on surgical wards? *Journal of Advanced Nursing*, 33(6): 728–37.

Seers, K. (1987) *Pain anxiety and recovery in patients undergoing surgery*, unpublished Ph.D. thesis, University of London.

Shi, S.F., Munjas, B.A., Wan, T.T.H., Cowling, I.W.R., Grap, M.J. and Wang, B.B.L. (2003) The effects of preparatory sensory information on ICU patients, *Journal of Medical Systems*, 27, 191–204.

Sloman, R., Rosen, G., Rom, M. and Shir, Y. (2005) Nurses' assessment of pain in surgical patients, *Journal of Advanced Nursing*, 52(2): 125–32.

Solomon, P. (2001) Congruence between health professionals' and patients' pain ratings: a review of the literature, *Scandinavian Journal of Caring Sciences*, 15(2): p174–80.

Squirrell, D.M., Majeed, A.W., Troy, G., Peacock, J.E., Nicholl, J.P. and Johnson, A.G. (1998) A randomized, prospective, blinded comparison of postoperative pain, metabolic response, and perceived health after laparoscopic and small incision cholecystectomy. *Surgery*, 123(5): 485–95.

Strong, J., Mathews, T., Sussex, R., New, F., Hoey, S. and Mitchell, G. (2009) Pain language and gender differences when describing a past pain event, *Pain*, 145(1–2): 86–95.

Tzeng, J.-I., Chou, L.-F. and Lin, C.-C. (2006) Concerns about reporting pain and using analgesics among Taiwanese postoperative patients, *The Journal of Pain*, 7(11): 860–6.

University of Texas MD Anderson Cancer Center (2009) *Symptom Assessment Tools: Brief Pain Inventory*. Available online at www.mdanderson.org/departments/prg/display.cfm?id=0EE7830A-6646-11D5-812400508B603A14&pn=0EE78204-6646-11D5-812400508B603A14&method=displayfull (accessed 1 July 2009).

Verbunt, J.A., Huijnen, I.P.J. and Köke, A. (2009) Assessment of physical activity in daily life in patients with musculoskeletal pain, *European Journal of Pain*, 13(3): 231–42.

von Baeyer, C.L., Spagrud, L.J., McCormick, J.C., Choo, E., Neville, K. and Connelly, M.A. (2009) Three new datasets supporting use of the numerical rating scale (NRS-11) for children's self-reports of pain intensity, *Pain*, 143(3): 223–7.

Warfield, C.A. and Stein, J.M. (1991) Psychologic factors, in C.A. Warfield (ed.) *Manual of Pain Management*, p. 16. New York: JB Lippincott.

Watt-Watson, J.H. (1987) Nurses' knowledge of pain issues: a survey, *Journal of Pain and Symptom Management*, 2(4): 207–11.

Wilson, G.A.M. and E. Doyle (1996) Validation of three paediatric pain scores for use by parents, *Anaesthesia*, 51: 1005–7.

Wright, K., Asmundson, G. and McCreary, D. (2001) Factorial validity of the short-form McGill Pain Questionnaire (SF-MPQ), *European Journal of Pain* 5: 279–84.

Further reading

Chapter 3, 'Assessment', in McCaffery, M. and Pasero, C. (1999) *Pain: A Clinical Manual*, CV Mosby Company, gives a useful overview of many of the problems encountered in clinical practice when assessing pain.

For a definitive and easy to understand overview of the MPQ, read the chapter on 'Assessment' in Melzack, R. and Wall, P.D. (1996) *The Challenge of Pain: A Modern Medical Classic*, Penguin Books.

The pharmacology of pain control

5

Chapter contents

Introduction
Mechanisms for drug action
Choice of analgesia
  Patient-related
  Drug-related
  Prescriber/dispenser-related
  Resource-related
  Legal and ethical issues
Drug effectiveness
  Absorption
  Distribution
  Metabolism
  Elimination
Drug delivery
  Compartments
Routes of administration
Different routes
  Rate of delivery
  Lipid solubility
  Calculating equivalencies ($\equiv$)
Plasma concentration

Duration of action
  Half life (t1/2)
  Repeat dosing
  Other factors affecting repeat dosing of
    analgesia
  Steady state
The three main groups of analgesics
  NSAIDs
  Paracetamol
  Opioid analgesics
  Other opioids
Other drugs used in the treatment of pain
  Anti-convulsants
  Anti-depressants
  Corticosteroids
  Local anaesthetics
  Capsaicin
  Cannabinoids
Summary
Reflective activity
References
Further reading

Introduction

One of the roles of the health care professional, as a member of the multidisciplinary team, is to work with the patient to devise a drug regime that reduces the patient's perception of pain to a minimum. The regime should support the patient's recovery and also maintain the mental and emotional well-being of the patient in chronic or terminal pain.

The choice of drugs available to alleviate pain is very wide and the selection of a particular drug in a particular patient or for a particular condition is governed by a number of factors including:

- the severity of the pain;
- the expected duration of the pain – whether it is acute short-term pain seen after surgery or an accident, or longer term as in chronic pain and cancer;

- the patient's previous response to analgesic drugs, particularly their tolerance to side-effects;
- the patient's emotional state and attitude to the cause of pain – this can be of paramount importance in chronic pain or the pain of terminal illness.

There are six broad areas that will be covered in this chapter. They are:

(1) mechanisms for drug actions;
(2) analgesic choice;
(3) drug effectiveness;
(4) routes of administration;
(5) duration of action;
(6) main groups of analgesics.

As a result the following objectives will be addressed:

- Demonstrate understanding of the main ways drugs act.
- Identify different routes of administration and their influence on the drug's action and effectiveness.
- Identify the three main groups of drug used in pain management: opioids, non-opioids and adjuvants.
- Be able to explain their mechanisms for action and how to utilize them effectively.

Mechanisms for drug action

Once a drug is administered and absorbed into the body it has to exert a pharmacological action before it is effective in relieving the patient's illness. Most drugs act by one of only three major mechanisms:

(1) *They replace or mimic the effects of a natural chemical messenger in the body:* an example of this type of activity would be the administering of morphine. Morphine replicates the effect of the body's own naturally occurring opioids – the endogenous opioid peptides (EOP).
(2) *They block or prevent the actions of a chemical messenger:* an example of this is administering adrenergic blocking drugs to block the effect of adrenaline in patients with heart disease. This results in a decrease in the work done by the heart.
(3) *They inhibit (and more rarely stimulate) enzymes:* an example of this type of action is the use of monoamine oxidase inhibitors to treat depression.

An understanding of how drugs act is useful when caring for individuals and when considering which drugs an individual is to be prescribed; it can be crucial in terms of the drug's intended effect and side-effects. For an easy digest on how drugs work in the body, the following is a useful source of information: www.doitnow.org/pdfs/223.pdf

More in-depth information can be obtained from the pharmacology texts included in the further reading section at the end of this chapter. Within this chapter, we only intend to address the pharmacology of pain and will be giving an overview of the main areas of importance.

Choice of analgesia

Choosing a painkiller for pain management depends on several different factors. These can be classified as:

- patient-related;
- drug-related;
- prescriber/dispenser-related;
- resource-related;
- legal and ethical issues.

Patient-related

There are several patient-related factors; four important ones are:

1. Drug acceptability.
2. Health problems that may prevent the use of a particular drug; for example, allergy or taking other drugs that interact with analgesia or an adverse medical history such as gastric ulceration or asthma.
3. Can they take the drug by a particular route?
4. Are they able to tolerate the effects of the drug?

Drug-related

Some of the important drug-related factors include:

- how easily the drug reaches the parts of the body it needs to get to;
- its ability to be given by a particular route;
- its duration of action;
- its metabolism and excretion.

Prescriber/dispenser-related

The prescriber is the person who decides which drug to give and the dispenser is the person who gives this drug to the patient. This might be the individual themselves; for example, if they are taking paracetamol at home. It might also be a doctor who prescribes and a nurse who dispenses in a hospital setting or if the doctor is a general practitioner who prescribes it could be the pharmacist who dispenses the drug. In all these cases there are some key elements that would influence the effectiveness of the drug:

- attitudes towards certain painkillers;
- beliefs about the strength or effects of certain drugs or routes;
- what the dose is and how frequently the drug is prescribed;
- how often the drug is given to, or taken by the patient.

Resource-related

Major factors here are:

- the cost of a drug;

- its availability, some analgesics are freely available; for example, from supermarkets, while others require a prescription;
- the way the drug is administered; an epidural analgesic will require far more resources than an oral analgesic.

Legal and ethical issues

Some painkillers have legal restrictions placed on them. In the UK many opioids come under the Controlled Drugs Act, which restricts their prescription and dispensing, while cannabis is illegal. This varies between countries; in the USA, for example, diamorphine, a commonly utilized opioid in the UK, is illegal and in the Netherlands, while cannabis is not legal, possession for recreational use is rarely prosecuted and for medical use is tolerated.

Drug effectiveness

The effectiveness of a drug depends on four factors:

1. absorption;
2. distribution;
3. metabolism;
4. elimination.

Absorption

When pharmacologists talk about the absorption of a drug into the body, they are describing the rate at which a drug leaves its site of administration (i.e. oral or injection) and the extent to which this occurs. For most routes it is unsafe to assume that 100 per cent of a drug will be absorbed. This can be particularly true after oral administration or the application of a drug to the skin in the form of a cream or ointment. In practice, providing we know how much is absorbed from a particular route and as long as individual drug responses do not vary greatly, all we need to really consider is the amount of drug that actually reaches its site of action.

Absorption is influenced by many factors. These include:

- *Drug concentration:* higher concentrations tend to be absorbed quicker.

- *The area of body surface available:* lungs have a large surface area available for drug absorption. Providing the concentration is correct, gases and vapours are absorbed at rates equivalent to an intravenous injection.
- *Formulation:* medicines that are already dissolved in solution are more rapidly absorbed than those given in the form of suspensions or capsules.
- *Chemical properties:* acids, such as aspirin, are poorly absorbed from the stomach as they are less soluble in the acid gastric juice. Many drugs are designed to be slightly acid so that they will be absorbed from the upper section of the small intestine and not the stomach.
- *Solubility:* whether a drug dissolves in lipids or in water will affect how rapidly it is taken up by the body's tissues as cell membranes have a lipid layer surrounding them. A lipid soluble drug gets to its site of action quicker but is also removed from the site more rapidly than a water soluble drug. See the section on 'lipid solubility' on p. 96.

Distribution

If drugs were transported in simple solution in the water of the blood plasma, they would be excreted rapidly by the kidney and their action would be of short duration. Instead, most drugs are bound loosely, and in a reversible manner, to plasma proteins. The drug bound to plasma protein is also in equilibrium with the unbound or 'free' drug in the plasma water, so binding acts as a reservoir from which the drug is released over time. It is important to appreciate that when a drug is bound to the plasma protein it cannot diffuse to its site of action, and therefore has no pharmacological activity. Only the small proportion of the drug that is free has any pharmacological activity or is available to be metabolized and eliminated. Plasma protein binding of drugs is therefore a major determinant in how long drugs remain active.

Plasma binding and drug toxicity

All drugs bind to the same sites on plasma proteins; as there are only so many sites available different drugs compete and this can lead to toxic interaction. Let us look at the mechanism of this interaction in a little more detail using the example of the anticoagulant drug warfarin and aspirin.

Warfarin is a useful drug in preventing vascular clotting in venous thrombosis and pulmonary embolism. It is also a toxic drug (it is used as a rat poison) which in overdose can result in bleeding into the joints and under the skin, leading to marked bruising. Normally doses are adjusted to ensure that plasma binding sites are not fully occupied providing a 'sink' to bind any slight excess of warfarin that may naturally occur. Also drugs which compete for these sites are avoided. About 99 per cent of warfarin is bound to plasma proteins; only one per cent will be in solution and pharmacologically active. As this 1 per cent is metabolized and excreted, more warfarin is released from the plasma protein, maintaining the ratio between bound and unbound warfarin and sustaining its therapeutic effect.

If aspirin is taken, the two drugs compete for binding sites and this displaces warfarin into solution so that the concentration of available warfarin rises. If it increases by just a few per cent then there is a danger of excessive bleeding. In severe cases, this may be fatal. This is why bleeding time in patients on warfarin is closely monitored.

Metabolism

> **Key point**
>
> The rate of metabolism is the main determinant of how long a drug will last in the body.

A drug's availability is primarily influenced by the way it is altered through the process of metabolism. Drugs are altered by enzymes in the tissue of certain organs, notably the liver, but drug-metabolizing enzymes are also present in the gastrointestinal tract, lung and kidney. The products of these enzymatic reactions (metabolites) usually behave differently to the original drug so that pharmacological activity can be:

- *decreased:* most metabolites are less active when compared with the original drug;
- *increased:* some drugs are converted in the body to the active compound, or the metabolite is more active than the original drug; such drugs are called pro-drugs;

Drug	Transformation	Action of metabolite
l-Dopa (inactive pro-drug)	Activation (in brain)	Dopamine (neurotransmitter)
Paracetamol	Oxidation (in liver)	Toxic metabolites
Amphetamine	Not metabolized	No change
Codeine	Metabolized to morphine	More active

Table 5.1 Some examples of altered drug activity

■ *unchanged:* a small number of drugs are not metabolized, but excreted unchanged.

Table 5.1 summarizes the activity of four drugs and their metabolites.

Drugs that are absorbed from the stomach or intestine pass through the liver before they reach the general circulation. The resulting metabolism inactivates most of the drug so that even if all of an ingested drug absorbs from the gut a significant proportion will be altered before it can reach its site of action. This decrease in bioavailability is called 'the first pass effect'. Most morphine-like drugs are considerably metabolized but in some this is an advantage. Codeine for example is metabolized into morphine while morphine is transformed into the metabolite *morphine-6-glucoronide* (M6G). M6G is an active metabolite and is more potent than morphine itself.

Elimination

The main route for drug elimination is through excretion by the kidneys but there are other pathways, such as the lungs, faeces and sweat glands. If there is disease or damage to the liver or kidney, the drugs or their metabolites are inefficiently eliminated; they may accumulate or duration of action increases.

It is important to know how much of the active drug is excreted unchanged because any change in the pattern of excretion due to disease or organ damage will have a profound effect on the therapeutic response to the drug. Clinical studies on healthy individuals indicate that 70 per cent of most drugs given intravenously are excreted unchanged (not metabolized) in the urine. This information is used to calculate how frequently a drug should be administered to maintain a consistent dose. Where there is impaired

kidney function, drugs are excreted at a slower rate, they remain in the body longer and the dose or the timing between two doses must be adjusted accordingly. Kidney function generally decreases with age and this means that different doses may need to be given to older patients.

Drug delivery

Compartments

A convenient way to think of drug delivery is to consider the body as being composed of a series of compartments.

Single compartment model

In a single compartment the drug simply needs to get into the plasma to work. An example of this is the use of normal saline for hydration. A simpler example is drinking water; we just have to drink it and it is absorbed into the blood stream across our gut. In the case of saline we bypass this process by cannulating a vein and putting fluid directly into the bloodstream. This very simple model depends on three factors, the amount of drug that can be absorbed, the degree of distribution around the body and the amount that is excreted. The first will be determined by the solubility of the drug and the second by the dose of the drug and the degree of first pass metabolism that occurs (see Fig. 5.1).

Two compartment model

In this model we have to consider that the drug not only has to enter the body but must also enter a target compartment to work and be reabsorbed from this to be excreted. We therefore have two compartments, the central compartment or plasma and a peripheral

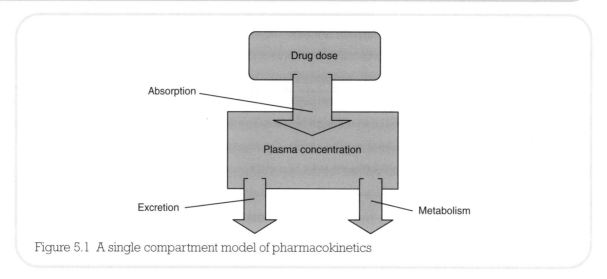

Figure 5.1 A single compartment model of pharmacokinetics

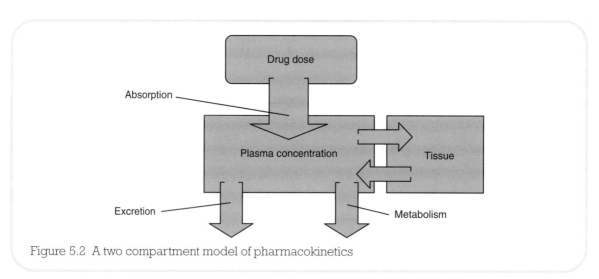

Figure 5.2 A two compartment model of pharmacokinetics

compartment representing the site of drug action. This closely approximates the action of non-steroidal anti-inflammatory drugs (NSAIDs) and paracetamol which work in the peripheral tissues, muscle, connective tissues, bones and skin. The time taken for the drug to arrive at, enter and leave the target tissue determines how long a drug will act and what concentration needs to be in the plasma. Plasma concentration levels therefore need to be maintained for enough of a drug to get to the target site (Fig 5.2).

Three compartment model

This model is helpful in considering the action of drugs that have to enter certain structures within tissues or where there are additional barriers in the way of a drug getting to its target. It helps to explain the action of opioids which act centrally, in the brain and spinal cord. These are protected by the meninges, a tough protective barrier consisting of three layers of lipid soluble tissue. Opioids, like other substances such as oxygen and glucose, have to diffuse across this barrier in order to reach opioid receptors in the central nervous tissue (see Fig. 5.3).

This adds an additional factor, getting into the central nervous system (CNS), which determines drug effectiveness and influences the duration and the necessary dose to ensure a sufficient plasma concentration.

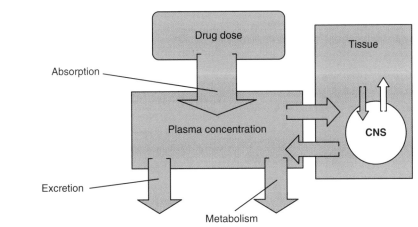

Figure 5.3 A three compartment model of pharmacokinetics targeting the central nervous system

Routes of administration

There are many different routes of administration for analgesia; Table 5.2 lists some of the most common ones. It should however be remembered that in most instances the best route for delivery of drugs is orally. This is not only a socially acceptable route for patients but is also a convenient and safe method for most drugs. Other routes are mainly of importance where the patient cannot swallow (McQuay et al., 1997) or if the pain is likely to be very acute and severe.

Oral	Rectal
Sublingual	Subcutaneous
Intramuscular	Intravenous
Epidural	Spinal or intrathecal
Topical	Transdermal
Buccal	Nasal

Table 5.2 Common routes used by analgesics

Different routes

All orally and rectally administered drugs are subject to first pass metabolism. This makes absorption inefficient and high doses are required when compared to parenteral (non-gastrointestinal) routes.

Buccal, sublingual, transdermal and nasal routes avoid first pass metabolism, so lower doses can be used. They still require absorption across a mucous membrane or the skin and the area of absorption is much smaller than the gut so the chosen drugs have to be very lipid soluble. Intramuscular and intravenous routes also avoid first pass metabolism and avoid absorption through skin or mucous membranes making them suitable for drugs that are weakly lipid soluble as well.

These routes all produce a global systemic effect as they must reach a sufficient plasma concentration to ensure that a drug reaches its target. They are effective at producing analgesia but expose patients to systemic side-effects as well.

Other routes target specific tissue sites. Topical applications attempt to do this, although as absorption is required across the skin, there is also a general systemic effect. Other methods of targeted administration include epidural, spinal and local infiltration (of local anaesthetics). These produce an effective response at a much lower dose and because of this avoid some systemic effects.

The suitability of a drug for a particular route depends on the rate of delivery required and its lipid solubility.

Rate of delivery

Gastric emptying and motility determine the rate of delivery of oral drugs to the small intestine where most absorption occurs. Absorption can thus be affected by the action of opioids like morphine on gastric emptying and motility. Because of this oral morphine is slowly and erratically absorbed. In severe acute pain, where rapid uptake is required, it is more effective if it is delivered intramuscularly or intravenously. An oral dose of morphine can take 90 minutes to be effective whereas an intramuscular dose may take 10–15 minutes and intravenously will be much quicker, less than five minutes. For chronic pains, however, slow release formulations overcome this erratic absorption by constantly releasing morphine into the gut.

Lipid solubility

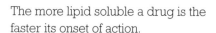

> **Key point**
>
> The more lipid soluble a drug is the faster its onset of action.

How quickly a drug can get across the lipid membranes of tissue will dictate its suitability for a particular route. For example, the opioid fentanyl is highly lipid soluble and is therefore suitable for administration in a transdermal patch. Morphine by contrast is weakly lipid soluble rendering it impractical for this route. To produce the same effect a huge transdermal patch, the size and volume of a backpack, with a very highly concentrated solution would probably be required. Morphine's relatively low lipid solubility is an advantage when given intrathecally as it will slowly pass through the arachnoid mater to enter the rich network of blood vessels in the epidural space and be transported away. This means that it will have a much longer duration of action than if given intravenously.

Calculating equivalencies (≡)

If a drug is administered by different routes into different compartments then its dose must be varied to avoid toxicity. Morphine is quite a convenient drug to

demonstrate this with. Calculating this dose adjustment involves working out the equivalent ratios of the drug in each compartment. Some texts refer to equivalencies as relative potency ratios.

As oral morphine absorption is affected by first pass metabolism a higher dose needs to be given than if the enteral route is avoided. A rough estimate is that the parenteral dose is equivalent to a third of the oral dose. If however morphine is delivered into the epidural space it only has to diffuse across the arachnoid membrane to reach the cerebrospinal fluid in the subdural space. It does not have to be distributed around the body before it comes into contact with the dura and therefore an epidural dose can be much lower to produce analgesia without any toxic effect. The actual dose need only be a tenth of the parental dose. Intrathecal (spinal) morphine however physically bypasses the arachnoid mater and is injected directly into the cerebrospinal fluid. As the morphine does not have to diffuse through the arachnoid membrane an even smaller amount of morphine is required. Once again the calculation for this is a tenth of the epidural dose.

> **Activity 5.1**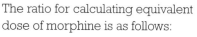
>
> The ratio for calculating equivalent dose of morphine is as follows:
>
> | | |
> |---|---|
> | Oral to parenteral: | 3:1 |
> | Parenteral to epidural: | 10:1 |
> | Epidural to intrathecal: | 10:1 |
>
> Calculate the following:
>
> 1 The intrathecal equivalent to 60 mg of oral morphine:
> 2 The oral equivalent of 5 mg of epidural morphine:
> 3 The intramuscular equivalent of 0.1 mg of intrathecal morphine

Your calculations *should have looked something like this*:

(1) The intrathecal equivalent is 0.2 mg of morphine. The calculation is as follows: 60 mg oral ≡ 20 mg parental ≡ 2 mg epidural ≡ 0.2 mg intrathecal.

2. The oral equivalent of 5 mg of epidural morphine is 150 mg. The calculation is: 5 mg epidural ≡ 50 mg parenteral ≡ 150 mg oral.
3. The intramuscular equivalent of 0.1 mg of intrathecal morphine is 10 mg as follows: 0.1 mg intrathecal ≡ 1 mg epidural ≡ 10 mg intramuscular.

What we are referring to here is the amount of a drug required to produce an effect at the target site. If we can reduce the dose that is given by directly targeting specific tissue, then we can reduce the dose of a drug and thus reduce its systemic effects. However, it should be remembered that this does not eliminate side-effects or risk of toxic effects as each equivalent dose is as potent as the next, and in certain cases such as intrathecal, because it is so close to the target tissue, may be even more likely to produce profound effects if dosing is not correct.

Plasma concentration

The graph shown in Figure 5.4 demonstrates the relationship between a drug's plasma concentration and its effect at its target site when a single dose is given.

From Fig. 5.4 you can see that to be effective a sufficient amount of drug has to be absorbed into the plasma. If too little is absorbed the drug has either no therapeutic effect or a short duration of action. The plasma concentration must be high enough to ensure that both an effective dose and duration of action is reached. For analgesics the dotted line representing the effective dose at target is known as the minimum effective analgesia concentration (MEAC) and is defined as 'the minimum plasma concentration at which analgesia occurs when a drug is given by constant infusion' (Charlton, 1997: 4)

Key point

The minimum effective analgesia concentration (MEAC) alters with pain intensity; this means that much higher doses are required for severe pain than for mild pain.

However, things are not that simple. Many analgesics when given in high doses have toxic effects. Morphine toxicity is first characterized by increasing drowsiness; this might be accompanied by

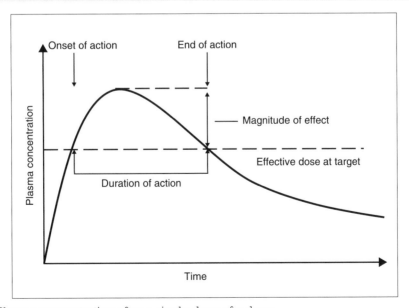

Figure 5.4 Plasma concentration after a single dose of a drug

a slightly reduced respiratory rate. As sedation increases the respiratory rate begins to slow down and the patient becomes unrousable. Pupils will become pinpoint, respiratory rate continues to diminish as respiratory depression progresses and eventually a respiratory arrest may occur and consequently death. It is important to differentiate between a toxic effect and a side-effect. Drugs like morphine have other effects such as nausea and vomiting or itching. Dysphoria, in the form of unpleasant visual hallucinations or nightmares, may also occur. These are unwanted side-effects as they occur at therapeutic levels and they can cause serious problems for patients. A very common side-effect is constipation. This occurs even at low doses of morphine and may be the reason for administering morphine in the first place as it is an effective anti-diarrhoeal medication.

When a drug is prescribed the dose has to be very carefully considered. There should be a sufficient dose to produce a therapeutic effect that has a good duration of action while avoiding too high a dose which will cause toxicity.

Duration of action

The margin between effective dosing and preventing toxicity restricts how much of the drug can be given. However, as soon as a drug is absorbed the processes of metabolism and elimination begin to clear it from the body. The initial concentration of the drug and its rate of clearance determine duration of action. In most drugs the clearance rate is proportional to the drug's concentration. This means that when there is a high concentration of the drug more is eliminated while when there is a lower concentration the rate of elimination is much slower. The result is a steady rate of reduction in plasma concentration of the drug known as the 'half life'.

Half life (t1/2)

Half life measures how long it takes for the concentration or amount of drug in the plasma to be reduced by exactly one-half. It depends on the drug behaving in a specific fashion known as a first-order reaction. If a drug behaves in this way then we know that the rate of elimination will follow a constant known as Kel for that drug. This is determined by the plasma clearance

and the volume of distribution (Vd) of a drug. Each drug has a specific Kel and t½.

If a patient cannot clear a drug from their body: for example, in liver disease where metabolism is reduced; in renal disease where elimination may be compromised; in the elderly who may not be as efficient in eliminating drugs because of loss of renal function; in the clinically obese where increased fat alters drug distribution; and in premature babies and neonates because their glomerular filtration rate is lower than normal adults; the Kel for the drug is altered and half life will be longer.

Conversely, in full term infants, renal function approaches young adulthood within one week of birth and doubles it by six months so that young children and older infants may well have a shorter half life for many drugs.

Activity 5.2

A patient is prescribed 20 mg of morphine. Morphine has a half life of approximately three hours. Calculate the amount of morphine still active at 24 hours after one dose of the morphine.

The answer is 0.078 mg of morphine. The calculation of half life is as follows:

$20 \text{ mg} \div 2 = 10 \text{ mg at 3 hours}$
$10 \text{ mg} \div 2 = 5 \text{ mg at 6 hours}$
$5 \text{ mg} \div 2 = 2.5 \text{ mg at 9 hours}$
$2.5 \text{ mg} \div 2 = 1.25 \text{ mg at 12 hours}$
$1.25 \text{ mg} \div 2 = 0.625 \text{ mg at 15 hours}$
$0.625 \text{ mg} \div 2 = 0.3125 \text{ mg at 18 hours}$
$0.3125 \text{ mg} \div 2 = 0.15635 \text{ mg at 21 hours}$
$0.15635 \text{ mg} \div 2 = 0.078125 \text{ mg at 24 hours}$

The above activity assumes that clearance is constant and not affected by clinical concerns and that the patient is a young adult.

Repeat dosing

Knowing the plasma clearance and half life of a drug is important when it comes to repeat dosing. Repeating doses before the half life has passed will increase a drug's plasma concentration leading to

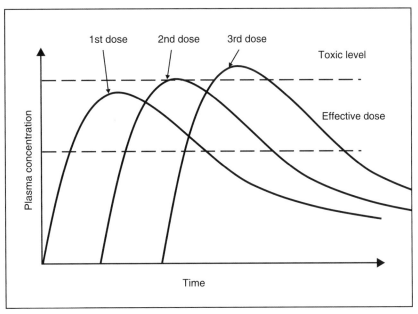

Figure 5.5 Repeat dosing before half life reached

toxicity. Where half life becomes extended due to health problems or age, toxicity can be a real problem unless the time between doses is increased (see Fig. 5.5).

In contrast, repeating doses after the half life means that the drug concentration will reduce and the level will fall below the minimum effective plasma concentration between doses. Where an analgesic is concerned this would mean a patient would experience pain in between doses (Fig. 5.6).

The graph of repeat dosing shown in Fig. 5.6 is commonly seen when analgesia is given to patients. Because the dose is repeated after the half life has passed, an analgesic's toxic effects are avoided and patient safety seems to be maintained. This can be a very important consideration when the serious and life-threatening toxic effects of many analgesics are concerned. It makes sense to protect patients from the adverse effects of a drug by ensuring the half life has passed before another dose is given. However, when the timing of the repeat dose is well past a drug's half life, a patient will experience unnecessary pain because the action of the first dose has long passed. We should also consider that aside from the ethical issues, pain itself, particularly acute severe pain,

causes adverse effects on a patient's health (see Chapter 7).

Activity 5.3

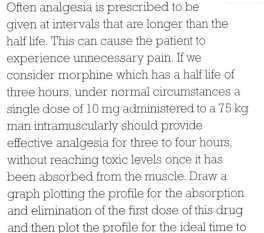

Often analgesia is prescribed to be given at intervals that are longer than the half life. This can cause the patient to experience unnecessary pain. If we consider morphine which has a half life of three hours, under normal circumstances a single dose of 10 mg administered to a 75 kg man intramuscularly should provide effective analgesia for three to four hours, without reaching toxic levels once it has been absorbed from the muscle. Draw a graph plotting the profile for the absorption and elimination of the first dose of this drug and then plot the profile for the ideal time to administer the second dose.

Your graph should resemble the one below (see Fig. 5.7). As you can see the three hour half life of morphine means that the patient can be kept safe and

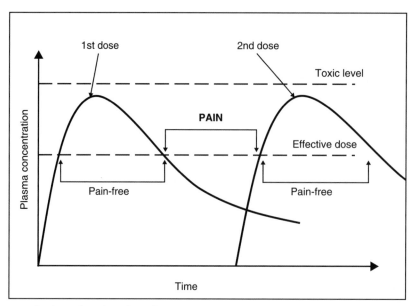

Figure 5.6 Repeat dosing of analgesia at intervals much greater than half life

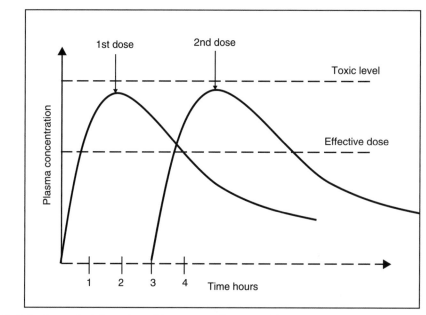

Figure 5.7 Pain-free administration of intramuscular morphine

quite comfortable as long as the dose is given every three hours.

Judiciously applying knowledge of the half life of a drug, its duration of action and the patient's health and age can reduce or eliminate the period of pain experienced between doses.

Reason	Explanation
Prescription is on demand	Carers do not actively assess pain and patients therefore have to request the analgesia and they only tend to do this when in pain
Many analgesics are controlled drugs	Controlled drugs are kept securely and must be checked and recorded in a controlled drug book by two members of staff. We audited how long this took. The quickest time was just over 15 minutes and the average was 45 minutes
The patient refuses the medication	When a painkiller is working, the patient is comfortable and often does not realize that the best plan of action is to anticipate the pain and repeat dose before it returns
The patient is asleep	It may seem cruel to wake someone in order to give them analgesia but in circumstances where they are likely to feel severe pain, taking analgesia by the clock will actually mean they experience more rest and less distress

Table 5.3 Other common factors affecting repeat dosing

Other factors affecting repeat dosing of analgesia

There are many other reasons why analgesics might not be given frequently enough to maintain the minimum effective analgesia concentration. Table 5.3 identifies some of the most common.

The optimum timing of a drug for repeat dosing should therefore ensure that the half life has passed but that the duration of action is maintained. That is, a balance between clearance and absorption occurs so that a high enough plasma concentration is maintained for effective analgesia without any toxicity. This balance is termed a 'steady state.'

Steady state

In activity 5.3 a steady state was achieved over two doses. However, Table 5.3 shows that organizational and other difficulties are likely to interfere with maintaining this over a long period of time. If a person requires long-term analgesia, then technical solutions can be used to maintain a steady state of a drug.

One such method is to use a continuous infusion of drug. In Figure 5.8 a graph represents a continuous intravenous infusion of morphine. In this example a steady state is achieved when the clearance rate and the infusion rate correspond. We can see that an initial peak occurs when the infusion commences and then

the drug begins to be eliminated. A problem with maintaining a steady state in many opioids is that the metabolites such as M6G are active opioids as well. These contribute to the effects of the drug and means that after a few hours toxicity will occur (see the dotted line) unless the infusion rate is adjusted. Maintaining a steady state using intravenous infusion requires regular and close monitoring for early toxic effects, such as drowsiness, with the infusion rate regularly adjusted.

Patient-controlled analgesia (PCA) is another technique which can produce a steady state if the patient is taught titration of their analgesia dose against their pain and this is covered in more depth in Chapter 7.

The three main groups of analgesics

The three main groups of analgesics are:

(1) NSAIDs;
(2) paracetamol;
(3) opioids.

NSAIDs

This is a diverse group of drugs that have different clinical structures but share similar therapeutic actions and side-effects (see Table 5.4). This makes it

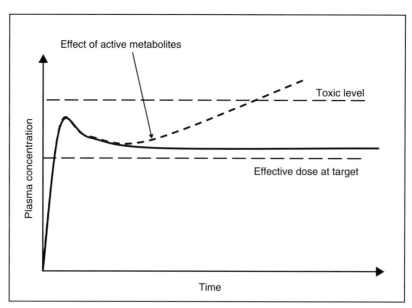

Figure 5.8 Steady state infusion of intravenous morphine

convenient to treat them together. Commonly used examples of these drugs are aspirin, diclofenac and ibuprofen.

NSAIDs' mechanism of action

The effect of NSAIDS and their side-effects arises from their ability to inhibit the enzyme cyclo-oxygenase, preventing the synthesis of prostaglandins from arachidonic acid. The prostaglandins are biologically active fatty acids involved in many physiological functions. One, P.G.E.$_2$, when synthesized in the brain, stimulates the hypothalamus to raise body temperature in fever. When it is synthesized in the stomach it reduces gastric acid secretion and increases gastric mucosal lining. Inhibiting this when pyrexic will reduce a fever; however, inhibition may also produce gastric ulceration. The adverse effects of NSAIDs on the stomach are more marked in elderly females. This is because oestrogen and progesterone have beneficial effects on the gastric mucosa and these hormones are lost after the menopause. Thinning of the gastric mucosa occurs in both sexes with age and

Action	Explanation
Anti-pyretic	Lowers body temperature in fever, has no effect on normal body temperature
Anti-inflammatory	They are powerful drugs in the treatment of conditions such as rheumatoid arthritis and osteoarthritis
Analgesia	Providing mild to moderate pain relief. More effective in headaches, bone pain and arthritis than visceral pain
Blood platelet aggregation inhibition	Aspirin is a first line of treatment for patients recovering from a heart attack and for prevention of a thrombosis in 'at risk' groups May produce dose-related gastric ulceration and bleeding

Table 5.4 Therapeutic actions and side-effects of NSAIDs

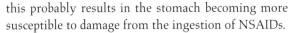

this probably results in the stomach becoming more susceptible to damage from the ingestion of NSAIDs.

Another, thromboxane, mediates platelet aggregation. Inhibiting this suppresses clotting. This is useful if you want to prevent thrombi formation but harmful if a gastric ulcer is present.

Prostaglandins are not stored within cells but are actively manufactured by a wide range of agents; at times of inflammation and tissue damage, they can be produced in excess and this leads to increased swelling, tissue damage and pain through the development of nociceptive hypersensitivity. These include, bradykinin, cytokines and Substance P. NSAIDs suppress the production of prostaglandin thereby disrupting this process and reducing stimulation of nociceptors.

Other side-effects

NSAIDs produce a variety of renal effects, including decreased renal blood flow and glomerular filtration. For this reason NSAIDs are contra-indicated or should be used with caution in patients with impaired renal function. Sodium retention can also occur, partly due to decreased glomerular filtration but also due to inhibition of renal prostaglandin synthesis, which augments sodium reabsorption. This can impact on hypertension, especially in the elderly who have reduced renal function.

In high doses NSAIDs also produce tinnitus and hearing impairment.

Drug interactions

NSAIDs are widely prescribed in the elderly for conditions such as osteoarthritis. However, this group of patients is also likely to have multiple health problems and may be taking several other drugs. Some particular NSAIDs have unique side-effects and interaction with other drugs. However, there is a wide range of drug interactions that can occur with any NSAID and it is always worth checking out interactions before commencing NSAIDs or using new drugs with existing NSAIDs. Earlier we considered interaction between warfarin and aspirin; this is seen in all NSAIDs. Other notable interactions are decreased renal clearance of digoxin and methotrexate, a commonly prescribed drug in rheumatoid arthritis.

Information required before starting treatment with NSAIDs

Before treatment starts you should check for contraindications. Common ones are haemophilia and gastrointestinal ulceration. However, breastfeeding and using aspirin in children is also contra-indicated, due to an association with Reye's syndrome.

Paracetamol

Paracetamol is not a NSAID although many of its actions are similar. It will reduce temperature in fever and is an effective analgesic but it does not have anti-inflammatory actions and only weakly inhibits cyclooxygenase. Although it does have a toxic metabolite it produces very few side-effects at normal doses, as this is quickly conjugated and bound with glutathione which neutralizes the metabolite. In higher than recommended doses however it can form a toxic metabolite which actively reacts with liver cells causing hepatic necrosis. Acute overdose may cause a fatal liver damage at a dose level of 10 g, which is two or three times the maximum dose of 4 g per day recommended for pain control in adults.

Opioid analgesics

The term 'opioid' is used to describe a group of drugs that are opium-like or morphine-like in their properties. These mimic the action of a group of natural substances called enkephalins, endorphins and dynorphins that act on the CNS to modify nociceptive pathways and reduce the sensation of pain. These are the endogenous opioid peptides and they are found in the brain and other areas of the body.

Mechanism of action of opioids

Opioids act centrally. They bind on opioid receptors within the CNS and throughout the body and have no action at the site of the pain. These receptors are binding sites for the naturally occurring opioids that suppress day-to-day aches and pains or are produced as a result of exercise. There are several opioid receptors including mu (μ), kappa (κ) and delta (δ) receptors. The most important for pain relief are the mu receptors. Opioid receptors are mainly located in the mid-brain and the posterior horn of the spinal cord.

When stimulated they suppress or inhibit pain transmission. Interaction with the receptors takes three forms:

1. *Stimulation:* this happens with many opioids such as morphine, diamorphine and pethidine – this is an agonist effect.
2. *The receptor is partially stimulated and partially blocked:* this occurs with buprenorphine – this is a partial agonist effect.
3. *The receptor is blocked:* this occurs with naloxone – this is an antagonist effect.

The mu (μ) receptor reduces the pain response through the CNS and produces the feeling of euphoria associated with this group of drugs. Unfortunately, this receptor also initiates a reduction in the carbon dioxide drive of the respiratory centre resulting in respiratory depression.

Properties of opioid-like drugs

Because all opioid-like drugs share a similar spectrum of pharmacological activity, we will look at the pharmacology of morphine in detail as a representative drug for the whole group. We will then mention one or two of the other drugs to indicate where they differ significantly in their effects from morphine.

Effects of morphine on the CNS

Morphine has the following effects on the CNS.

In severe pain it produces analgesia and increased tolerance to pain. For this reason opioids like morphine are the first line treatment for severe acute pain (McQuay et al., 1997). At higher doses, drowsiness, euphoria and mental clouding can occur. Other sensations such as touch are not affected so pain can still be located but perception and emotional stress are reduced.

In the majority of pain-free individuals the administration of morphine produces dysphoria, anxiety and vomiting.

In high doses, morphine produces marked constriction of the pupil of the eye – miosis – through CNS stimulation. Pinpoint pupils can be taken as a diagnostic sign of overdosage and can be seen before respiratory depression becomes apparent.

Morphine is a powerful respiratory depressant.

When given to people who are not in pain or in doses larger than required to control the pain – as may occur in pains that are non-responsive to opioids – morphine acts on the respiratory centre in the medulla oblongata to reduce its responsiveness to carbon dioxide. Opioid responsive or nociceptive pain probably inputs into the respiratory centre and as a result death from an overdose of morphine is normally the result of respiratory depression.

Use of morphine in the short term, for acute pain, does not affect the production of endogenous opioid peptides. Longer-term use in chronic pain or palliative care will suppress endogenous opioid peptides; this may lead to increased opioid tolerance requiring dose increases and difficulty in withdrawal because of existing pain.

Opioid addiction occurs in individuals who have no pain but abuse opioids; there is no evidence that appropriate medical use of opioids for nociceptive pains produces drug-seeking behaviour associated with illicit drug use (McQuay, 2008).

Effects on the gastrointestinal tract – long-term use

Morphine has the effects on the gastrointestinal tract shown in Table 5.5.

Effects on other smooth muscle

Morphine has a dual effect on the bladder, increasing detrusor muscle tone, producing a feeling of urinary urgency while also increasing sphincter tone, making voiding difficult. Tolerance to this effect develops but it can lead to retention of urine. Morphine can also prolong labour by affecting the uterus.

Other effects of opioid-like drugs

- Cough inhibition through suppression of the cough reflex.
- Biphasic effect on body temperature. Low doses decrease body temperature; higher doses increase body temperature.
- Histamine release – in the bronchioles the release of histamine can cause bronchoconstriction. This, combined with the respiratory depression produced by morphine, can make breathing difficult. In the skin, morphine can cause dilation of the

Effect	Mechanism
Constipation	Inhibition of inte... decreased gas... transit time wh... reabsorption...
Decreased secretion of hydrochloric acid in the stomach and biliary, pancreatic and intestinal enzymes	Delayed food...
Constriction of the Sphincter of Oddi	Causes an ir... Patients with biliary cone... may... increase rather than a decrease in pain when given opioids

Table 5.5 Effects of morphine on the gastrointestinal tract

surface blood vessels leading to flushing. Also, the release of histamine in the skin can produce pruritus or itching.

Therapeutic action of opioids

As you have seen, opioids have widespread pharmacological actions. Three major therapeutic uses for opioids are as follows:

1. analgesia;
2. controlling diarrhoea;
3. cough suppression.

Adverse reactions

Earlier in this chapter we discussed the toxic effects of morphine and we differentiated these from its side-effects: Some of the commonest side-effects that can occur at therapeutic doses include:

- *Constipation:* this occurs, to a greater or lesser extent, in most patients receiving these drugs. The use of regular prophylactic laxatives is therefore always indicated when opioids are administered.
- *Respiratory depression:* this is also common. It is dose-dependent and results from depression of the respiratory centre in the medulla oblongata.
- *Nausea and vomiting:* on first-dose administration, morphine stimulates the chemoreceptor trigger zone in the medulla oblongata to produce a feeling of nausea and even vomiting. In most

patients this effect is not seen on subsequent administration.

Other opioids

Other opioids display the same characteristics as morphine with variations in their lipid solubility, half life and effect at receptor sites that may make them more useful than morphine in certain clinical situations.

Diamorphine (heroin)

Diamorphine is modified from morphine. Its analgesic potency is three times greater than morphine's. It has a more rapid onset of action but a shorter duration of action. In the UK it is the drug of choice for subcutaneous administration due to its high water solubility. This permits the administration of high concentrations of the drug in a small injection volume. Diamorphine is a very powerful drug of dependence. Its manufacture, sale and use, even in clinical situations, are illegal in the USA. Diamorphine is normally used when morphine is ineffective in pain control.

Diamorphine is particularly useful to relieve the acute pain of myocardial infarction and left ventricular failure when pulmonary oedema is present. Diamorphine depresses the exaggerated effects of respiratory effort, reduces patient distress and anxiety and helps to redistribute blood volume to the peripheries. Diamorphine is also less likely to induce nausea and vomiting.

...he alkaloids present in opium. Its ...effects are similar to morphine, with ...th of its potency. Much of its effect ...partial conversion to morphine in the liver. ...nately, approximately 10 per cent of the ...ation are lacking the enzyme responsible for this ...version.

It is also an excellent cough suppressant and produces less respiratory depression than morphine and has a lower abuse potential. Low-dose preparations are available as over-the-counter medicines combined with many other pharmacological agents to assist its analgesic properties.

Pethidine

Pethidine is an older synthetic drug that is used as both an analgesic and an antispasmodic. It has a shorter half life than morphine, approximately two hours. Pethidine has been advocated as a drug with a reduced effect on smooth muscle in comparison to morphine. Consequently, it has been and still is advocated for hepatic and renal colic and in surgery in these areas, such as cholecystectomy or for acute management of pancreatitis, although the evidence base is inconclusive in supporting this.

Pethidine has one distinct disadvantage to morphine. Its metabolite norpethidine has a longer half life than pethidine and duration of action than morphine and when given in repeated doses or to patients with impaired renal function, it will accumulate and irritate the CNS and can cause convulsions.

Pethidine is widely used for occasional administration during labour. Its shorter half life may mean that the mother is able to metabolize more of the drug and that less crosses the placenta to have an effect on neonatal respiration. However, there is no evidence for this and the use of pethidine in labour in the UK continues, as a tradition, mainly because it is a drug that midwives are allowed to prescribe and administer.

Mixed agonist/antagonist opioids

These drugs were developed in an attempt to produce morphine-like analgesic drugs which do not produce euphoria and which are therefore less liable to abuse. In varying degrees they share all the pharmacological effects of morphine, such as analgesia, respiratory depression, cough suppression, nausea and vomiting.

Methadone

Methadone is more effective after oral administration than morphine and has a longer duration of action but about the same potency. The major difference between morphine and methadone is that methadone is synthetic and does not produce as much euphoria. It also suppresses the withdrawal symptoms characteristic of opioid drug dependence and blocks the euphoric effect of heroin and morphine. Both tolerance and physical dependence can occur with methadone as with most opioids, but these are less severe.

Fentanyl

Fentanyl is a synthetic morphine-like drug but with considerable higher potency. Its use during induction of anaesthesia allows a reduction in the anaesthetic drugs but requires care due to the high risks of respiratory depression. It has a relatively long half-life lasting – about 6–8 hours – although in the elderly this may increase to 15 hours. Fentanyl is useful in anaesthesia as it has a rapid onset and is also used transdermally in palliative care because of its higher lipid solubility.

Tolerance, dependence and withdrawal symptoms

In pharmacological terms the three characteristics of tolerance, dependence and withdrawal seen in opioids relate to different aspects of their action as drugs and are not adverse effects or side-effects. However, these characteristics are often linked together and are commonly confused.

Tolerance

Tolerance to the pharmacological or therapeutic effects of a drug is a widespread phenomenon. It is seen in situations where increasing concentrations of the drug have to be given to maintain the same level of efficacy or effectiveness as originally seen with a lower dose. It does not occur where a patient's condition is deteriorating and they report an increased severity or intensity of pain which requires an increase in dose. It occurs because the metabolism of the opioid increases due to enzyme activity in the liver, making less of the drug available in the first place or because the nervous system adapts to the concentration of opioids by producing more opioid receptors so that the drug is utilized more rapidly or reduces the production of endogenous opioid peptides requiring more of the administered drug to be used for background purposes. This may be dealt with either by dose escalation or changing the opioid or the route.

Dependence

Dependence refers to a state of physiological adaptation, with the patient needing to use the drug to prevent withdrawal effects. The risk of drug dependence is low in the therapeutic use of opioids; when the pain ceases patients no longer require analgesia. Dependence is often erroneously confused with addiction which describes an abusive pattern of behaviours that may or may not be driven by physical or psychological dependence that can be described as an overwhelming and compulsive need to use the substance of abuse.

Withdrawal symptoms

If opioids are suddenly withdrawn from a tolerant individual then within one or two hours the individual starts exhibiting withdrawal symptoms. Such symptoms include:

- dysphoria and increased sensitivity to pain and touch;
- increase in secretions from nose, mouth and gastrointestinal tract;
- diarrhoea and severe intestinal cramps;
- widely dilated pupils;
- respiratory and cardiovascular stimulation.

The severity of the withdrawal symptoms can be reduced or abolished by withdrawing the opioid slowly through gradually reducing the daily intake.

Other drugs used in the treatment of pain

In palliative care and neuropathic pain management a small number of drugs, which are not classified either clinically or pharmacologically as analgesic drugs, are used for pain relief. Why such drugs should act as analgesics in some patients is not always clear, and their use in palliative care often involves non-licensed indications, routes and dosages. Not all patients respond to these drugs and they are always introduced into treatment as an adjuvant after treatment when powerful drugs such as morphine have failed to provide complete pain relief for the patient. When the decision has been made to use adjuvant drugs, the starting dose should be low and the patient should be carefully monitored. These include:

Anti-convulsants

Anti-convulsant drugs are useful in some types of neuropathic pain. Until recently there has been no drug of choice but carbamazepine and sodium valproate are commonly used. However, in the elderly, anti-convulsant drugs used in relatively high doses can produce sedation and dizziness. Two drugs that have been shown to be efficacious in neuropathic pain even in these vulnerable groups are gabapentin and pregabalin. They are now the drugs of first choice.

Anti-depressants

Tricyclic anti-depressant drugs such as amitryptiline and nortryptiline have also proven useful as an adjutant in neuropathic pain. As with the anti-depressant action of these drugs, it takes seven to ten days after treatment before any therapeutic effect becomes noticeable. They do have uncomfortable side-effects and these can quite often be hard to tolerate and are the main cause of non-concordance. If patients can be persuaded to persist for a few weeks then these side-effects tend to diminish and the pain-relieving properties can be appreciated. A beneficial side-effect is drowsiness and for this reason they are prescribed at night to help with sleep. Nortryptiline is better tolerated than amitryptiline and a related drug imipramine has only mild effects but is less effective as an adjuvant.

Corticosteroids

Patients with bone pain can obtain additional pain relief by using steroids such as dexamethasone as an adjutant.

Local anaesthetics

Local anaesthetics act by reversibly blocking peripheral nerve impulses. They inhibit sodium influx and hence nerve membrane depolarization so nerve transmission is inhibited. They affect autonomic, sensory (pain, temperature, touch and pressure) and motor fibres depending on the drug and concentration used and where they are placed. Local anaesthetics are used to infiltrate wounds during surgery as well as in epidural analgesia solutions but are short-acting drugs.

There are two groups of local anaesthetics.

1. Amides, which are mostly injected, for example, bupivacaine and lignocaine, metabolized by liver.
2. Esters, which are mostly topical such as cocaine, procaine, metabolized by tissue esterases.

The potency of local anaesthetics is related to lipid solubility and the effect on the vascular system. All clinically used local anaesthetics cause vasodilation with the exception of cocaine which is an intense vasoconstrictor and is restricted in use both because of its addictive effects and the fact that prolonged use will produce tissue ischaemia. The vasodilatory effects are an important consideration in the management of epidural analgesia.

Some of the side-effects of local anaesthetics are listed below although these are not particularly common and mainly occur as a result of accidental intravenous injection during epidural anaesthesia when excessive plasma concentration results in CNS and cardiovascular system (CVS) toxicity.

- *CNS stimulation:* apprehension, anxiety, restlessness, confusion and disorientation.
- *CNS depression:* drowsiness and respiratory arrest.
- *CVS:* local anaesthetics are anti-dysrhythmic agents and can depress contraction of cardiac muscle causing hypotension and cardiac arrest and dysrhythmias.

Capsaicin

Capsaicin is derived from the chilli pepper. It is used as a rubefacient and acts peripherally on C neurones and thinly myelinated Aδ neurones to block conduction if used regularly in high doses topically in the painful area. Capsaicin has been supported by research for use in a number of pain disorders, both nociceptive and neuropathic. For example, rheumatoid and osteoarthritis, post-herpetic neuralgia, stump pain and post-surgery scar pain and diabetic neuropathy. It may need to be used for 1–2 weeks before pain is relieved. Its main side-effect is an intense transient burning sensation during initial treatment, particularly if too much cream is used, which reoccurs on subsequent treatment if the frequency of administration is less than 4–6 hourly.

Cannabinoids

Like opium, cannabis contains many substances that have effects on the CNS. Some of these have been demonstrated to have an anti-nociceptive effect through blocking specific cannabinoid receptors.

Currently, the use of cannabinoids for pain in the UK is restricted to specific research projects and is under Home Office licence. Recent advances include evidence that cannabinoid agonists are anti-hyperalgesic and anti-allodynic in neuropathic pain. Development of novel cannabinoid agonists and cannabinoid preparations that are anti-nociceptive has important implications for the therapeutic use of this class of drug. It is widely used as an analgesic by many people with chronic pain. This is currently illegal in the UK and in addition poses additional health problems. There is some evidence that users of cannabis in its natural rather than in a medicinal form who smoke the drug are more likely to develop respiratory diseases than people who smoke tobacco because they smoke it without a filter, and it has been linked with mental illness in chronic users.

Summary

Having briefly examined the mechanisms for drug action, this chapter explored the absorption, transport, metabolism and elimination of drugs and explained how these properties impact on the drugs' ability to fulfil their action. The last section of the chapter has explored the analgesic effects of many of the drugs commonly prescribed in practice. The nature and actions of the drug have been considered together with what drugs should be prescribed in a variety of different patient scenarios.

For a more detailed account of their actions refer to the further reading section at the end of this chapter.

From the areas we have explored you should be able to:

- understand the main ways drugs act;
- identify the main routes of administration;
- relate routes of administration to action and effectiveness;
- identify the three main groups of analgesic drugs;
- explain the main functions of non-opioid drugs;
- explain the main mechanisms of opioid drugs;
- discuss the use of adjutant drugs.

Reflective activity

As a conclusion to this chapter consider how knowledge of this theory will help you in your future practice. Try to be specific and use the following points/questions as a guide.

- *State* which elements of the chapter will help you in your future practice.
- *Elaborate:* be specific in terms of how this knowledge and understanding can be used in practice.
- *Give examples:* of care events which would benefit from what you have learnt.
- What are the *implications* if you change the way you practise.

You may prefer to use a reflective model such as Gibbs's (1988) to guide your reflection (see Appendix at the end of this book). Think of a specific example as the starting point; for example, a patient's pain management where an opioid had been prescribed. When analysing the situation draw on this chapter's theory to support your discussion and demonstrate your understanding. As a result of your reflection you should evaluate:

- the appropriateness of the drug prescribed;
- the impact of the dose, route and frequency on the effect and side-effects exhibited by the patient.

References

Charlton E. (1997) The management of postoperative pain, *Update Anaesthesia*, 7(2):1–7.

McQuay H. (2008) *Opioid Use in Chronic pain* available online at www.medicine.ox.ac.uk/bandolier/booth/painpag/wisdom/S31.html (accessed 20 July 2009-07-21).

McQuay, H., Moore, A. and Justins, D. (1997) Treating acute pain in hospital, Fortnightly review, *British Medical Journal*, 314: 1531.

Further reading

British National Formulary (date unknown) BNF online at www.bnf.org/bnf/

Brody, T.M., Larner, J. and Minneman, K.P. (1998) *Human Pharmacology: Molecular to Clinical*, 3rd edn. Edinburgh: Mosby.

Downie, G., MacKenzie, J. Williams, A. (2008) *Pharmacology and Drug Management in Nurses*, 4th edn. Edinburgh: Churchill Livingstone.

Galbraith, A., Bullock, S., Manias, E., Richards, A. and Hunt, B. (2007) *Fundamentals of Pharmacology: A Text for Nurses and Health Professionals*, 2nd edn. Harlow: Pearson Education Ltd.

Gibbs, G. (1988) *Leaving by Doing: A Guide to Teaching and Learning Methods*. Oxford: Further Education Unit, Oxford Polytechnic.

Greenstein, B. and Gould, D. (2009) *Trounce's Clinical Pharmacology for Nurses*, 18th edn. Edinburgh: Churchill Livingstone.

Hopkins, S.J. (1999) *Drugs and Pharmacology for Nurses*, 13th edn. Edinburgh: Churchill Livingstone.

Prosser, S., Worster, B., MacGregor, J., Dewar, K., Runyard, P. and Fegan, J. (2000) Applied *Pharmacology: An Introduction to Pathophysiology and Drug Management for Nurses and Healthcare Professionals*. Edinburgh: Mosby.

6

Delivering pain management

Chapter contents

Introduction
The organization of pain management
Development of chronic pain services
The palliative care service
The acute pain service (APS)
Patient education
   Difficulty in understanding
   The knowledgeable patient
Risk management
   Patient-related risks

Capacity
Intellectual capability
Identifying and managing potential
   complications
Drug effects
Problems with epidurals
Staff support and development
Summary
Reflective activity
References

Introduction

This chapter focuses on the organized provision of pain management using pain management services. We briefly touch on the history and structure of acute pain, chronic pain and palliative care services before moving on to the function and purpose of these services. We focus on the acute pain service (APS) as much of the research into delivery of pain management focuses on this particular area and using examples we explore how the pain service can be structured to enable improvements in technological methods, such as epidural- and patient-controlled analgesia (PCA), and care to be safely developed and delivered.

There are four broad areas covered in this chapter. They are:

1. the organization of pain management;
2. patient education;
3. risk management;
4. staff support and development.

As a result the following objectives will be addressed:

- How to deliver safe and effective pain management within an organization.
- How to support patients and staff using pain management techniques.

The organization of pain management

Pain is increasingly recognized as a problem in its own right rather than as a symptom of other diseases. This, accompanied by the development of pain management as a speciality in its own right, has led to significant improvements in the quality of pain management and innovation in methods of treating, alleviating and managing pain. The formation of pain management services within health care organizations has driven this development. Such services offer a systematic and logical approach to the provision of pain management and this has built up an evidence base on the best methods for managing pain and provides support and structure to the delivery of pain management. These have been advocated as a means to manage pain for a number of years (Mann and Carr, 2008). The first pain management services were set up in the 1940s and 1950s (Meldrum, 2003) and initially focused on chronic pain and palliative care in the UK. Although palliative care services dealt with more than pain they did bring to bear a whole systems approach to the problems which eventually influenced other types of pain management services. Both these services were led by charismatic figures, such as Dame Cicely Saunders in the UK and Dr John Bonica in the USA, who advocated a multidisciplinary and multiprofessional approach to pain management. However, the reality was that historically these services arose locally out of a special interest rather than any coherent strategic planning.

Development of chronic pain services

The first chronic pain services started in the 1940s as a means of providing pain relief through specific interventions such as anaesthetic blocks and sympathectomies. They were invariably performed by a single anaesthetist and some of these developed their expertise so that they were regularly referred patients and were able to establish clinics (Clinical Standards Advisory Group, 2000). This has led to mixed and patchy provision although the ideal pain clinic is defined by the Audit Commission (1997) as the fully multidisciplinary clinic. In the UK, the Association of Anaesthetists of Great Britain and Ireland and the Pain Society (1997) recommended, as a minimum standard, that every chronic pain treatment centre should have access to 'multidisciplinary' resources for appropriate patients while their preferred approach is through a multidisciplinary clinic. In 1997, this was the least common in the UK (see Table 6.1); the most common being the partially multidisciplinary anaesthetist-led clinic with a third as anaesthetist-only services. However, provision of chronic pain services is very variable. Some populations had no local access and workloads in clinic can vary by as much as 10-fold (Dr Foster, 2003).

The Dr Foster (2003) report largely reviewed the situation regarding specialist chronic pain clinic services available in UK hospitals. It showed that there have been improvements in some areas and worsening in others, but that chronic pain services are still highly variable across the country. For example, multidisciplinary clinics have increased slightly, but

Fully multidisciplinary	Clinics staffed by anaesthetists and doctors from several other specialities, plus other specialist staff (e.g. nurse, psychologist, physiotherapist, pharmacist)	Uncommon
Partial multidisciplinary 1	Anaesthetist-led with a doctor from at least one speciality, plus other staff	20% of clinics
Partial multidisciplinary 2	Anaesthetist-led with at least one other non-medical specialist member of staff (usually a nurse or physiotherapist)	40% of clinics
Single discipline	Anaesthetist-only service	33% of clinics

Table 6.1 Variations in staffing of chronic pain services
Source: Audit Commission (1997, Table 3: 85.)

there are less pain clinics available and while quality improvements have occurred, there is still patchy provision and long waiting times as well as a lack of emphasis on early treatment and possibly preventative measures in primary care.

The palliative care service

Although pain management is a very important function of the palliative care service, it is not their only function. In the past palliative care grew out of the treatment and management of cancer at the end stages of life and dealt with all the symptoms that arose as a result of the process of dying. Now it often aspires to deal with any progressive life-threatening disease, although its core condition remains cancer. This is because palliative care services tend to be seen by health care providers as exclusive to people who are in the late stages of terminal cancer and there is significant voluntary provision provided by cancer specific charities, so that the needs of people with other conditions are neglected or subsumed into services oriented towards cancer care (Small and Rhodes, 2000). A 'palliative approach' that aims to provide both physical and psychosocial well-being is an essential part of professional care (Bach, 1998). This is necessary as the majority of people with cancer experience moderate or severe pain and other symptoms (WAG, 2003) and 'most of these symptoms can be controlled through adequate care with a palliative approach.' It is when a patient's distress shows no sign of improvement that referral to specialist palliative care is required. This puts a strain on organizations as palliative care crosses institutional boundaries (Clarke and Seymour, 1999).

It has been recommended that palliative care services are used in four ways:

1. to give advice and information to professional colleagues, with no contact with an individual patient;
2. to make a one-off consultative visit to a patient, then advise the team;
3. to offer short-term interventions for specific problems, then withdraw;
4. to offer ongoing, multiple problem-solving advice and intervention, with regular assessment (Glickman, 1996).

The acute pain service (APS)

The acute pain service originated in the USA but in the UK an influential report by the Royal College of Surgeons of England and Royal College of Anaesthetists (1990) led to an increase in services for patients with acute pain after surgery in the UK. The goal of this report was to improve the patient experience of acute pain after surgery. Prior to the development of the APS pain relief after surgery was haphazard and often criticized for *'poor prescribing and administration habits, poor assessment of pain, lack of awareness of the problem and the general inflexibility of the hospital organisation'* (Pediani, 1998: 154). The APS has also developed for other reasons including a better understanding of pain science, recognition that pain management has therapeutic as well as a humane and moral value and a drive to improve the quality of care for patients after surgery.

It is no coincidence that the development and growth of PCA and then epidurals as methods of postoperative pain management accompanies the development of the APS. The two are closely linked as many services started out as a means of monitoring and evaluating the effectiveness of these technical means of analgesia, which involved giving control over potentially lethal drugs to patients and using expensive equipment. It was a reciprocal arrangement as new techniques required the development of the APS, their existence increased the use of PCA and epidurals through providing safer environments for them to operate in. This helped overcome fears and resistance, so that they are now viewed as ordinary and not extraordinary practice. The principles established by the development of what were often at first PCA services provide a good platform for the development of other techniques.

The structure of an APS varies between organizations but it tends to be multidisciplinary involving a team approach that usually has anaesthetists, a specialist nurse and a dedicated pharmacist at its core (Bäckström and Rawal, 2008; Mann and Carr, 2008). The role of the service tends to consist of:

- monitoring the efficacy of pain management; for example, through audit;
- offering advice and support to other staff and patients;

- troubleshooting difficult problems and intervening to provide direct care; for example, epidural 'top-ups';
- education and development of staff in acute pain management;
- standardizing treatment and prescriptions so that all carers know what normal practice is;
- where non-standard measures are required, providing direct care and support to ensure safe practice;
- controlling the use and distribution of technical and expensive equipment, such as PCA devices and epidural pumps.

Often the member of the multidisciplinary team who is either responsible for these activities or whose role is to coordinate them is the specialist nurse (Alexander and Williams, 2009). Increasingly, APSs have been involved in additional perioperative care issues such as nutrition, hydration and prevention of complications (Carr and Mann, 2000) and they have been used as a starting point for the development of more comprehensive critical care outreach services (Aneman and Parr, 2006). Often the APS focuses on post-surgical pain, either because of constraints on resources or organizational difficulties (Audit Commission, 1997). Areas of acute pain management that might not be directly served by an APS include: accident and emergency departments, coronary care units, medical wards, outpatients, primary health care, follow-up of patients discharged from day surgery, elderly care and the elderly mentally ill (Clinical Standards Advisory Group, 2000). A useful activity would be to find out whether or not the APS in your locality addresses pain issues in these areas.

We consider the main duties of an APS to be the improvement of post-operative pain management through the better use of existing methods and the introduction and promotion of new methods of managing pain. This must be supported by the education and training of those who provide care to surgical patients and the development of guidelines and protocols for them to follow. Additionally, the APS must monitor compliance to these sets of rules through audit and other means of quality control including selection, purchase, and the supply and maintenance of suitable equipment. Last, but not

least, the APS should be involved in research at some level.

In an attempt to bring these three types of service together, the Association of Anaesthetists of Great Britain and Ireland and the Pain Society (1997) recommended the ideal structure for a pain management service as an integration of acute and chronic pain and cancer-related symptom control with the responsibility and the provision of such an integrated service shared across various interests and specialities within an overall coordinated structure. Over the past 12 years there have certainly been improvements in organization and communication between the three types of pain service but an overarching structure has rarely been developed. It seems that pain services can be isolated within an organization, not engaged with wider objectives or activities and have difficulty communicating with health professionals not directly involved in the services (Powell et al., 2009). Yet each of these three services, if successful, is based on the following three foundations: patient education, risk management and staff support and development, all of which should be the concern of any health care organization.

Key point

Whatever their nature, pain services need to adopt a systematic, structured and multidisciplinary approach if they are to be effective.

Activity 6.1

In order to find out about how a pain service operates you can contact your local pain management team and ask them the following questions.

1. Is the pain service integrated or separated into acute, chronic and palliative care services?
2. Is the service multidisciplinary? Who are the members of the pain management team?
3. What activities is the pain service involved in?

(4) What groups of patients does the pain service look after? For example, does a palliative care service only look after cancer patients or does an APS only provide care to surgical patients?

Patient education

Patient education is an important health intervention that can be used to empower patients, through information-giving, fostering choice and raising awareness and promoting self-control over their condition (Johansson et al., 2003). In pain management it often involves teaching, counselling and behaviour modification with the aim of encouraging patient participation in their care as well as reinforcing the therapeutic relationship (Schrieber and Colley, 2004). Often patient education is preplanned and focused on delivering specific content but it can also occur in an *ad hoc* fashion that focuses on issues as they arise. Both approaches can be effective as long as they combine the evidence base with clinical expertise (Johansson et al., 2003). In this way difficulties in understanding can be overcome and patients can become knowledgeable.

Difficulty in understanding

The key to successful and safe pain management is to ensure the patient understands what is required of them. For example, in an acute pain setting this might mean they should understand how to operate a PCA device. This requires explanation and instruction and depends on the patient's mental capacity. Anxiety and fear may be confounding factors but good patient education can generally overcome these. Where this is not possible or where someone does not have capacity then avoid using PCA; this is easy to do when you already know someone suffers from dementia but harder when they develop post-operative delirium, although this can be screened (Sly-Havey, 2009). We should however be sure of diagnosing confusion as can be illustrated by Case study 6.1 which recounts one of the author's experiences of dealing with a patient who developed sedation problems because they did not understand PCA.

Case study 6.1

While working as an acute pain nurse one of the authors (Parsons) was called to see a patient who was 'getting confused and disoriented and was alternatively very drowsy and then very aggressive and abusive' and was now doubly incontinent as well, with a request to change her analgesia regime to IM injections as it was 'obvious that the PCA did not agree with her'.

On going to the ward to assess the patient he found a distressed lady who was upset that the nurses were ignoring her when she requested a bedpan and was very angry that she had ended up soiling herself. She was pain-free and coherent, just very upset and annoyed and convinced that the nurses were neglecting her.

As we were talking she decided to call the nurses to tell them off again. She picked up a handset to do so, but instead of this being the nurse call button, she pressed the PCA button. It was obvious what the problem was. In her ignorance of how a PCA operated she had confused the PCA demand button for the nurse call button and was using this to call the nurses to get her a bedpan.

Of course as they were not responding to her demands, she pressed the PCA button more and more; a situation that safety features, such as lock-out and dose limit, would not remedy as she was pain-free when she pressed the button. As a consequence she had been giving herself too much morphine and would fall asleep. The PCA device showed that she had made over 1000 demands in the previous 12 hours. After doing this several times she eventually soiled herself and took exception to being 'neglected' by the nurses and wanted to tell them off – hence her 'abusive behaviour'.

A simple explanation of how the PCA worked and showing her the difference between the nurse call button and the PCA button was all that was required to resolve the problem. The patient was not confused but misinformed.

Confusion and misinformation over pain management can mean that care is ineffective with patients either experiencing unnecessary pain or experiencing adverse events such as excess sedation, as in this case. When such problems arise it is not a reason to avoid introducing effective pain management, it just requires more care and attention.

The knowledgeable patient

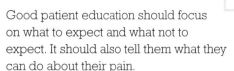

Key point

Good patient education should focus on what to expect and what not to expect. It should also tell them what they can do about their pain.

A pain management technique requires patients to be knowledgeable and supported in order to get the best use of the method of managing their pain. This applies as equally to technical devices, such as a PCA, as it does to behavioural modification techniques such as cognitive behavioural therapy (CBT). These involved a detailed explanation, preferably delivered by a knowledgeable professional prior to use. In the case of PCA this might be an anaesthetist or an accredited registered nurse. For a technique such as CBT this might be some other member of the multidisciplinary team, such as a clinical psychologist or a physiotherapist. These explanations should involve the following: a practical demonstration, discussion of benefits and potential adverse effects, including drug side-effects, strategies for dealing with these and an opportunity to express concerns (Sherwood, 1996).

In the case of PCA, the explanation was based on the evidence derived from early studies which focused on reducing analgesia consumption and pain experience through promoting targeted drug delivery. The purpose was to address concerns expressed by health professionals that PCA use produced higher consumption of opioids than conventional 'as required' intramuscular injections (Shade, 1992). It ignored the probability that in the past under-medication significantly contributed to post-operative pain. This approach heavily emphasized pre-operative preparation, instilling patients with a theoretical under-

standing of PCA and giving strict instructions on what to do, specifically when and how to demand a dose. In acute pain a similar approach was also adopted for teaching patients about epidural analgesia, with an emphasis placed on physical aspects, including; how the epidural is inserted, positioning on insertion, how their pain will be assessed and why they are being monitored, what the effects of the different drugs used are and explaining technical terms such as *height of block* and why they might need to have a urinary catheter (Strathern, 1996).

In acute pain this approach is now criticized as more recent evidence demonstrates that structured approaches to patient education do not improve overall analgesic efficacy or pain scores significantly in patients who have a PCA, although initial satisfaction with the method is better (Lam et al., 2001). Instead, other measures are more important, including continuing education and post-operative supervision by the acute pain team. The researchers suggested that pre-operative PCA education only produced short-term and transient gains and that the ongoing experience is more important. This is supported by later work by Chumbley et al. (2004) who re-examined the same questions asked by Shade (1992). In this large study the effectiveness of information delivered in two ways, by a patient-determined leaflet or an interview by a trained nurse from the pain team, were compared to a control of normal pre-operative information. They demonstrated that patients in the leaflet group were better informed, less confused, and more capable of using the PCA than the control group or the group interviewed by the acute pain nurse. There were also no significant differences in pain relief, worries and knowledge of side-effects between the three groups. These are criteria that in our opinion would affect satisfaction. These findings suggest that providing detailed pre-operative information by acute pain nurses is not economical in terms of producing benefits for the patient using a PCA although the use of information leaflets can provide good support.

More recently Kastanias et al. (2009) identified that adults undergoing surgery were extremely interested in information about their likely pain experience after surgery and were specifically interested in what they could do to manage their pain and how to deal with adverse effects, such as nausea, rather than worrying about fear of addiction. Of particular interest was information on what pain to expect after discharge and what to do about it.

Our opinion is that while information leaflets provide important information, education involves more than this. It also involves understanding what to do when they are in pain. In the case of technical methods, this may involve how to use the equipment and reinforcing technique once the device is up and running, but in other areas it may be reinforcing and modelling good behaviours, such as administering analgesia by the clock, rather than waiting for pain to become a problem. In this regard the role of the ward nurse is vital, as they should strengthen apposite practices.

We also consider that an emphasis on pre-operative information-giving is not the best use of the acute pain team's time. This is because it only focuses on delivering information at one given point of time and one that seems to us to be packed with all sorts of sensory and cognitive information that may flood a person's senses and will therefore impair learning. Instead, we believe that the team's focus should be ensuring ward nurses are appropriately educated and supported in the provision of ongoing education to patients as this is a much more effective strategy. In this way it is possible to: ensure the right patient is selected; assess their competence; reassure the patient about what is normal and what is abnormal; and reinforce patient safety; for example, in the case of PCA giving information such as 'only you should push the demand button'. This means of course that an APS cannot control the fine detail of patient education but should have systems in place that enable those in regular contact with patients, that is, the ward nurses can educate, support and inform patients (Breivik and Stubhaug, 2008). Such systems should include not only what to teach patients but also how to teach patients and we would advocate a person-centred approach which emphasizes individual needs rather than one that focuses on delivering predetermined information (Edwards, 2009). It should be remembered that learning depends on attitude and motivation and the possession of relevant previous knowledge and experience (Johansson et al., 2003).

Risk management

Risk management incorporates several factors; some of these relate to the patient, some to the organization and some to the specific technique used to manage pain.

Patient-related risks

Patient suitability

A method of pain management may not be suitable for all patients. Some are at particular risk of experiencing side-effects and others may be unable to use the technique. For example, in acute post-operative pain management, PCA is useful where people are unable to take oral medication or where their pain is likely to be severe enough that they require strong doses of parental opioids as an alternative to frequent intermittent intramuscular or intravenous injections. However, some patients who meet these criteria are not suitable. These include those who are physically or mentally incapable of using the device; have impaired consciousness; have difficulty in understanding the concept of PCA; have a severe respiratory problem; or suffer from obstructive sleep apnoea. Another category includes patients with severe pain who are cared for in areas with a high nurse to patient ratio as these are likely to have a continuous intravenous opioid infusion. Finally, some patients would prefer some other method of pain control and are unwilling to use PCA.

Another technical method of pain management, continuous epidural analgesia, involves an invasive procedure that is not without risks to the patient or client either in pain or at risk of developing pain. Where epidurals are used effectively they can give significant benefits but they are not suitable for all. Williams and Wheatley (2000) indicate three groups of people who might benefit from epidurals. These are those:

(1) who cannot use intravenous PCA;
(2) who are undergoing major surgery such as: major joint replacement, upper abdominal surgery, caesarean section, thoracotomy or lower body vascular surgery; that is, those who have a greater risk of experiencing surgical stress;
(3) who have other medical problems which preclude them from safely having a general anaesthetic,

such as chronic obstructive airways disease or heart failure.

Enabling choice

There are times when a person's choices are limited. For example, in an emergency hip operation in a frail elderly person, an epidural may be the only option for their anaesthetic if they want the operation to proceed. This will provide pain relief during surgery, but they will always have a choice as to whether or not they use an epidural for pain relief after this period. This is more than an issue of obtaining informed consent. If a patient is anxious about a particular pain management technique they might still consent because logically they can see it makes sense even though they are emotionally horrified at the prospect. Ideally, any patient should be happy with their choice as this will ensure that they benefit psychologically as well as physically from their chosen method of pain management. Some of the ways of helping patients become happier involve:

- making sure that decisions about pain management are patient-centred; that is, the patient is at the heart of making the decision and feels in control of the process;
- discussing the effects and side-effects as part of giving information prior to consent but also detailing how they are going to be protected from these side-effects;
- previous contact with the clinician or therapist who will be delivering the technique, and related to this:
- developing a positive therapeutic relationship;
- respecting concerns as real and valid and adapting pain management plans around this; for example, avoiding acupuncture in someone who is needle-phobic;
- identifying what is normal and what is abnormal.

For example, it is important to explain to patients what they will experience. With an epidural, if they are prepared to expect some weakness in their limbs or a loss of proprioception then they are unlikely to be distressed by it. However, if the aim is to achieve a sensory block without motor block, if patients cannot move their lower limbs they need to be told to inform nursing staff as this might indicate that the block is too strong. Conversely, pain sensation would indicate that the block is too weak. Similarly, when a patient is prescribed a trycyclic antidepressant as an adjunctive analgesic, they should be warned that it takes time to become effective, they are likely to experience a dry mouth and may temporarily get blurred vision and that they could feel drowsy. Otherwise, they will feel that their new drug is not relieving their pain and that they are just experiencing side-effects.

Capacity

Physical capability

The fundamental idea of a method of pain management like PCA is that the patient is capable of demanding a dose. If someone other than the patient uses the device, then this is no longer 'patient-controlled' analgesia, it is pain relief by some other means and a key safety feature has been removed, exposing the patient to a greater risk of sedation and respiratory depression. Obviously, PCA requires patients to operate the device themselves as they must be physically capable of demanding a dose. Most devices use a handheld push button to achieve this but there are commercially available alternatives, foot pads and squeezable appliances. It is important to avoid assumptions about physical capability; however, consider the comment from a patient with a congenital deformity of their hands in the following Case study (6.2).

Case study 6.2

. . . because I have no fingers or thumbs it was just assumed that I wouldn't be able to use a PCA device and I was given injections for pain in my leg. But it was no good and I hurt so much that I couldn't stand it and complained. After the pain team came, I was able to show that I could use the PCA by trapping the button under my chin and since I've started using the pain machine, things are much better.

A common form of physical incapacity is state of consciousness, just as a sedated patient will not demand a dose from the PCA a patient with impaired consciousness is physically incapable of operating the device.

Intellectual capability

Loss of consciousness is also a form of intellectual capability and the capacity to understand and therefore consent to pain management is certainly an important right. However, people with intellectual incapacity, such as those with some learning disabilities (Donovan, 2002) or with dementia, are a very vulnerable group whose pain is often inadequately managed (Zwakhalen et al., 2007) mainly due to deficits in knowledge and assessment. Even where intellectual capability is impaired it is still possible with care to use demanding techniques; for example, the use of PCA should not automatically be precluded from those patients who have a learning disability. An individual assessment to ascertain the nature and extent of their learning disability is required in this vulnerable group (Davies and Evans, 2001). Even with a relatively severe learning disorder good use of PCA can be achieved (Case study 6.3).

> **Key point**
>
> The decision to use a particular technique should involve an individual assessment of capability.

Identifying and managing potential complications

Problems with the pain management technique

Problems can arise from using a particular technique, either because of error or failure in the technique or because the technique has intrinsic properties that are

---

Case study 6.3

Angela Davies was undergoing surgery to correct a joint deformity in her hip (a hemiarthoplasty) and was therefore likely to experience severe pain. She was living in supported accommodation and her registered learning disability nurse, Peter, accompanied her. Angela had a moderately severe learning disability (Down's syndrome) and was unable to give informed consent. But she was able to communicate well with Peter and could make her wishes known. She was less communicative with most of the ward nurses but seemed to form a close attachment to one of the student nurses (Helen) on the ward.

To support Angela, the APS was involved in drawing up a pain management plan. Angela was to have a general anaesthetic and then an epidural for post-operative pain management: Peter and Helen carefully explained this to Angela and she was happy to agree to this. Unfortunately, the epidural was unsuccessful, although it was possible to administer spinal morphine. Instead, Angela had a prescription for intramuscular morphine. One of the reasons for deciding on an epidural in the original management plan was that Angela was very frightened of injections and it quickly became apparent that this was a wholly inappropriate prescription.

The ward nurses called the acute pain team and a PCA device was set up with specific instructions for the nurses to give her a bolus dependent on a safety assessment of Angela's respiratory rate and level of sedation. This was set up in order to provide some pain relief with the acknowledgement that, given her level of understanding, it would be unlikely to produce effective pain management. However, Angela was interested in the device and Helen, the student nurse, spent considerable time teaching her how to use the demand button appropriately. Angela proved perfectly capable of deciding to press the button when she had pain and needed a little prompting in order to anticipate pain. This was a valuable lesson for all the staff involved.

risky and need to be managed. Where a technique is applied and it fails to relieve pain, then a patient has been exposed to a risk without receiving the required benefit. This should be avoidable but often, particularly in chronic pain management where there may not be a suitable pain-relieving technique available, it might arise that a method is chosen that is controversial because there is not a consensus on its suitability or the long-term risks are unacceptable to some. An example of such a controversy is the use of opioids in chronic pain which according to Littlejohn et al. (2004) is shaped more by concerns about iatrogenic addiction than their actual efficacy. In their conclusion they:

> . . . suspect that, as happened previously with acute pain and palliative care, fears about addiction from opioid therapy in chronic non-cancer pain have been excessive. This is not to argue that opioids are always the drug of choice for chronic pain – just that excluding them a priori appears based more upon ignorance than on science.
>
> (Littlejohn et al., 2004: 64)

The decision whether to use opioids is based on the prescriber's judgement of relative risks. Some techniques that hold potential risks are worth doing because, when successful, they have a profound benefit – through relieving pain or preventing other complications. Continuous epidural analgesia is a good example of this. The occurrence of pain while an epidural is in place can be said to be a failure of the technique or its ongoing administration and care. Failure rates among epidurals for post-operative pain quoted in the literature are very wide from as little as 2 per cent to as much as 23 per cent (Kumar and Smith, 2003). That there is such a wide variation in failure rate must relate to more than just the technique but to the organization and delivery of the technique as well. Epidurals are a tricky procedure and there are several reasons why they may fail to produce an adequate analgesic block (see Table 6.2).

We would assert that the role of a pain management service is to minimize such risks; in this case through a mixture of quality control and education of those inserting and maintaining the catheter.

Drug effects

The various drugs that are commonly used to manage pain also have intrinsic risks and can produce side-effects such as:

- respiratory depression;
- nausea and vomiting;
- excessive sedation;
- confusion and hallucinations;
- pruritus (itching);
- hypotension;
- constipation.

For example, opioids like morphine act primarily on the body's μ receptors and despite having a desired analgesic effect can also contribute to several unwanted effects that need to be monitored and

Failure	Possible reason
No analgesic block	The catheter: wrongly positioned or movement from original position, or has fallen out (5–25% of incidences (Kumar and Smith, 2003)
	The epidural pump has failed
	The infusion rate is inadequate
	Drug dose inadequate
Patchy or partial block	Catheter is inserted too far or not far enough so all affected dermatomes are not covered
	Position of the patient has altered the distribution of the epidural solution, e.g. lying on one side for a long time

Table 6.2 Reasons why an epidural block might fail

managed differently depending on the setting, and although they occur in most situations will therefore require different prioritization for monitoring and prevention.

Problems with epidurals

Epidurals use a mixture of local anaesthetics and opioids and have additional side-effects due to the fact that a nerve block will produce paraesthesia in the area supplied by the nerves affected. As the spinal nerves pass through the epidural space they are bathed in the local anaesthetic. Spinal nerves are composed of both efferent nerves, for example, motor nerves supplying skeletal muscles, and afferent nerves supplying peripheral information. Both types of nerve are affected resulting in both a motor block, which is not desired, and a sensory block, which is. The effect is differential as the sensory nerve fibres affecting nociception are thinner than other sensory and motor fibres and many are unmyelinated. The thickness of a neurone and the presence of a myelin sheath protects a nerve against a local anaesthetic, thus sensory nerves are affected before the thicker and heavily myelinated motor nerves. A physiological phenomenon that is useful therapeutically in ascertaining sensory block without causing undue pain is the fact that cold sensation is blocked at the same time as pain sensation, because it is also conducted by some of the nociceptive fibres and travels along the same spinothalamic tract in the cord as pain messages. As a consequence, ice is used to identify the presence and extent of sensory block. Light touch and pressure sensation is affected in a similar way as is proprioception.

As well as an unwanted motor block, the sympathetic nervous system (SNS) which runs in parallel to the spinal cord is also blocked. Among other actions the SNS stimulates the heart beat, maintains a normal tone in blood vessels and responds to low blood pressure by producing vasoconstriction in the skin and viscera, thus maintaining and raising blood pressure and decreasing gut motility. A SNS block prevents these actions and unless compensated for gives rise to some of the adverse effects that can occur with epidurals. Blocking the heart is not usually a problem in therapeutic levels of epidural analgesia as the sympathetic nerves supplying the heart leave the epidural

space at T1 and T2 and although it may in theory occur in high thoracic epidurals or when an epidural block gets too high, the authors have been unable to find any case evidence in the literature.

A far more common problem is the vasodilatating effect of the epidural block; some vasodilatation is inevitable in a local anaesthetic blockade and has to be compensated for in some way. The effect is dependent on both dose and spread of the epidural, so in stronger concentrations of local anaesthetic and larger epidural blocks the risk is greater. This is a common occurrence with a range from 3–30 per cent of epidurals (Williams and Wheatley, 2000) and if not compensated for the patient becomes vulnerable to hypotension. This effect is even more pronounced in individuals with impaired cardiovascular performance, particularly a history of arterial hypertension, and if other vasodilators are given to the patient, for example, sublingual glycerine trinitrate (Klasen et al., 2003). There are measures that can be taken to counter this which include preloading with intravenous fluids prior to injecting the infusate, close monitoring of fluid balance to avoid depletion, and ensuring the block is maintained so that top-up boluses are not required.

Trim et al. (2003) discuss how they adopted a clinical governance approach to the problems they encountered with epidurals in their pain management service. Essentially, they perceived problems in those areas that did not follow set guidelines and standardized practices for epidural care; this occurred for various reasons. Clinical governance is a quality approach to managing health care based around evidence and accountability for action. Trim et al. (2003) utilized audit and a review of the evidence base to identify deficiencies in the epidural service and improve the quality of care received by patients on epidurals. A major problem was the use of variable rather than a standardized prescription mix of local anaesthetic and opioid.

Key point

All pain interventions have risks; good pain management requires you to balance these risks against any benefits.

Staff support and development

It can be seen that epidurals and other pain management techniques have risks that need to be balanced against their benefits by good supporting actions by a pain management service. These actions aim to reduce operator errors, problems arising from the specific technique, mismanagement, the priority given to pain management and communication errors. These are all organizational factors and they can be divided into three categories – for the purposes of our discussion, we continue with the use of epidurals as an example, because this is an area that has received a lot of attention, but the underlying principles apply to all methods of managing pain.

(1) *Competence* To provide safe care requires knowledgeable practitioners (Royal College of Anaesthetists et al., 2004). Obviously this has major implications as to how and where you can provide care for a person in pain. It follows that if you want to provide a quality service then any area whether it is a critical care setting, a general surgical ward, a clinic, or the community should have competent care providers. Competency involves both knowledge and experience. The development of this competency is a major function of pain management services and is achieved through a mixture of competency identification, standard setting, training, education and supervision.

(2) *Workload* There is a wide distribution in the location where patients with epidurals are cared for (Minzter et al., 2002) but all require patients to be safely monitored and observed and for this to happen there has to be sufficient suitably trained and educated people, usually (but by no means exclusively) registered nurses, available to do this correctly (Royal College of Anaesthetists et al., 2004). Often an organization has guidelines in place that set out minimum acceptable requirements and to safely care for a patient in a particular location these must be met. This influences how many people can have a particular intervention. For example, if a hospital restricts patients with continuous epidural analgesia to a high dependence area, this may prevent other patients from using these services or prevent high-risk patients who require an epidural from having surgery in the first place. This will influence the choice of technique available and may contribute to selection of a method that has fewer risks but is not as effective. Schafheutle et al. (2001) surveyed nurses to answer the question 'Why is pain management suboptimal on surgical wards?' A third of respondents cited a lack of time to perform duties, including monitoring because of workload issues as a significant factor in suboptimal care.

(3) *Technical support* Technical support can be considered to involve the following: support for clinical care, including help available for troubleshooting and clinical emergencies; auditing the quality of care provided and recommending improvements; ongoing support for professional decision-making; the development of clinical skills and knowledge; supply and delivery of materials; and support for device purchasing and maintenance.

The key elements in dealing with organizational issues have been identified by (Idvall et al., 2002) (see Table 6.3).

Element	Content
Communication	Informing and educating, routines and teamwork
Action	Detecting and acting on signs and symptoms, acting on behalf of patients
Performing	Specific care and general care: prescriptions and techniques
Promoting	Relationships and trust; competence, knowledge and appropriate attitudes
Environment	Protecting patients and staff and providing equipment

Table 6.3 Key elements in dealing with organizational issues
Source: Idvall et al. (2002)

Idvall et al. (2002) used these elements in a quality performance tool designed to evaluate acute pain management services. This tool breaks each category into several quality indicators. If we look in detail at Idvall et al.'s (2002: 534) last category, the quality indicators for 'environment' include the following statements:

"over half the caring staff on the ward must be registered nurses"

"there must be special rules for the documenting of pain assessment and treatment"

"nurses must possess special knowledge of pain assessment and pain treatment"

"there must be a particular nurse who is responsible for the individual patient's pain treatment (a primary nurse)"

Activity 6.2

If you agree with Idvall et al.'s (2002) tool, which is based on published guidelines on optimum pain management care that have been published by expert groups, such as the American Pain Association, you might like to consider a clinical environment you work in and whether the above four factors apply using the following questions:

1. What is the ratio of registered nurses to unregistered carers in this clinical area?
2. Are there guidelines on the documentation of pain assessment and treatment?
3. Have nurses had education and training in pain assessment and treatment?
4. Is there an individual nurse who is responsible for an individual patient's pain treatment?

This obviously has major implications as to how and where you can nurse a patient in pain if you want to provide good quality, and thus by implication safe care. A standard has been set that the minimum level should include more than 50 per cent of carers who should be registered nurses and these should:

- possess theoretical and skills-based knowledge of epidurals;
- be prepared to take responsibility for the treatment a patient receives;
- follow written guidelines for the management of epidurals.

It might be the case that the clinical area you have considered does not meet the environment standards proposed by Idvall et al. (2002). This does not necessarily mean that the care delivered in these areas is not of a reasonable quality but it does mean that different judgements will have been made that it is safe to send patients with advanced pain management techniques, such as PCA or epidurals, to a clinical area. It would be an interesting exercise to consider whether such judgements are based on a logical reasoned approach arising out of evidence. Remember in Chapter 6, we asked you to consider whether expert judgement is the best form of evidence and in this chapter we have discussed how other approaches, for example, Trim et al. (2003) identified different approaches to evaluating the quality of a pain service.

Summary

Throughout Chapter 6 we have considered some general principles regarding the role of pain management services. In particular we have considered issues around patient selection, equipment, safety, education and training. There needs to be several systems in place to promote effective pain management and while there will always be a variation between organizations key principles include:

- good communication between all concerned parties;
- selection of appropriate patients;

- controlling who does what: for example, only designated competent people set up and manage a particular technique;
- standardization of method: for example, using standard prescription guidelines, with clear instructions given, in order to avoid drug errors and a method for recording variations from the norm;
- professional education systems that incorporate assessment, recognition and minimizing side-effects, troubleshooting, what to do and who to contact if help is needed;
- audit and other methods of quality control;
- openness to evidence-based ideas and if possible opportunities to perform research.

Reflective activity

As a conclusion to this chapter consider how knowledge of this theory will help you in your future practice. Try to be specific and use the following points/questions as a guide:

- *State* which elements of the chapter will help you in your future practice.
- *Elaborate:* be specific in terms of how this knowledge and understanding can be used in practice.
- *Give examples:* of care events which would benefit from what you have learnt.
- What are the *implications* if you change the way you practise.

You may prefer to use a reflective model such as Gibbs's (1988) to guide your reflection (see Appendix at the end of this book). Think of a specific example as the starting point; for example management of PCA in your clinical area. Describe the event and then proceed through the cycle. When analysing the situation draw on this chapter's theory to support your discussion and demonstrate your understanding. As a result your reflection should examine the key principles included in the Summary's bullet list.

References

Alexander, S. and Williams, C. (2009) Nursing accountability for pain management: working within an in-patient pain service, *Pain Management Nursing*, 10(1): e3.

Aneman, A. and Parr, M. (2006) Medical emergency teams: a role for expanding intensive care? *Acta Anaesthesiologica Scand*, 50: 1255–65.

Association of Anaesthetists of Great Britain and Ireland and the Pain Society (1997) *Provision of Pain Services*. London: Association of Anaesthetists of Great Britain and Ireland and the Pain Society.

Audit Commission (1997) *National Report: Anaesthesia Under Examination*. London: Audit Commission.

Bach, I. (1998) Specialist palliative care services: all Wales minimum standards 1998. Draft report, Holme Tower Marie Curie Centre, Penarth.

Bäckström, R. and Rawal, N. (2008) Acute pain service – what it is, why it is and what is next? *European Journal of Pain Supplements*, 2(1): 40–3.

Breivik, H. and Stubhaug, A. (2008) Management of acute postoperative pain: still a long way to go! *Pain*, 137(2): 233–34.

Carr, E.C.J. and Mann, E.M. (2000) *Pain: Creative Approaches to Effective Management*. Basingstoke: Macmillan.

Chumbley, G.M., Ward, L., Hall, G.M. and Salmon, P. (2004) Pre-operative information and patient-controlled analgesia: much ado about nothing, *Anaesthesia*, 59(4): 354.

Clarke, D. and Seymour, J. (1999) *Reflections on Palliative Care*. Maidenhead: Open University Press.

Clinical Standards Advisory Group (2000) *Services for Patients with Pain*. London: Department of Health.

Davies, D. and Evans, L., (2001) Learning disability nursing: assessing pain in people with profound learning disabilities, *British Journal of Nursing*, 10(8): 513–6.

Donovan, J. (2002) Learning disability nurses's experiences of being with clients who may be in pain, *Journal of Advanced Nursing*, 38(5): 458–66.

Dr Foster (2003) Adult chronic pain services in the UK. Report by Dr Foster in consultation with the Pain Society.

Edwards, S. (2009) Patient education: educating patients and families about their surgery, *Journal of PeriAnesthesia Nursing*, 24(3): e6.

Gibbs, G. (1988) *Learning by Doing: A Guide to Teaching and Learning Methods*. Oxford: Further Education Unit, Oxford Polytechnic.

Glickman, M., (1996) *Palliative Care in the Hospital Setting*. London: National Council for Hospice and Specialist Palliative Care Services.

Idvall, E., Hamrin, E. and Unosson M. (2002) Development of an instrument to measure strategic and clinical quality indicators in postoperative pain management, *Journal of Advanced Nursing*, 37(6): 532–40.

Johansson, K., Leino-Kilpi, H., Salanterä, S., Lehtikunnas, T., Ahonen, P., Elomaa, L. and Salmela, M. (2003) Need for change in patient education: a Finnish survey from the patient's perspective, *Patient Education and Counselling*, 51(3): 239–45.

Kastanias, P., Denny, K., Robinson, S., Sabo, K. and Snaith, K. (2009) What do adult surgical patients really want to know about pain and pain management? *Pain Management Nursing*, 10(1): 22–31.

Klasen, J., Junger, J., Hartmann, B., Benson, M., Jost, A., Banzhaf, A., Kwapisz, M. and Hempelmann, G. (2003) Differing incidences of relevant hypotension with combined spinal-epidural anesthesia and spinal anesthesia, *Anesthesia and Analgesia*, 96(5): 1491–5.

Kumar, N. and Smith, G. (2003) Postoperative pain: inpatient in D.J. Rowbotham and P.E. MacIntyre (eds) *Clinical Pain Management: Acute Pain* Chapter 16 London: Arnold.

Lam, K.K., Chan, M.T., Chen, P.P. and Kee, W.D. (2001) Structured preoperative patient education for patient-controlled analgesia, *Journal of Clinical Anesthesia*, 13(6): 465–9.

Littlejohn, C., Baldacchino, A. and Bannister, J. (2004) Chronic non-cancer pain and opioid dependence, *Journal of the Royal Society of Medicine*, 97(February): 62–5.

Mann, E. and Carr, E. (2008) *Pain Creative Approaches to Effective Management*, 2nd edn. Basingstoke: Palgrave Macmillan.

Meldrum, M.L. (2003) A capsule history of pain management, *Journal of the American Medical Association*, 290(18): 2470–5.

Minzter, B.H., Johnson, R.F. and Grimm, B.J. (2002) The practice of thoracic epidural analgesia: a survey of academic medical centers in the United States, *Anesthesia and Analgesia*, 95(2): 472–5.

Pediani, R.C. (1998) Organizing acute pain management, in B. Carter (ed.) *Perspectives on Pain: Mapping the Territory*, Chapter 12. London: Arnold.

Powell, A.E., Davies, H.T.O., Bannister, J. and Macrae, W.A. (2009) Challenge of improving postoperative pain

management: case studies of three acute pain services in the UK National Health Service, *British Journal of Anaesthesia*, 102(6): 824–31.

Royal College of Surgeons of England and Royal College of Anaesthetists (1990) *Report of the Working Party on Pain after Surgery*. London: RCS/RCA,

Schafheutle, E.I., Cantrill, J.A. and Noyce, P.R. (2001) Why is pain management suboptimal on surgical wards? *Journal of Advanced Nursing*, 33(6): 728–37.

Schrieber, L. and Colley, M. (2004) Patient education, *Best Practice & Research Clinical Rheumatology*, 18(4): 465–76.

Shade, P. (1992) Patient-controlled analgesia: can client education improve outcomes? *Journal Advanced Nursery*, 17(4): 408–13.

Sherwood, K. (1996) *Patient Controlled Analgesia Booklet*, Australia: Ryde Hospital.

Sly-Havey, M. (2009) Using the dementia quick screen to predict post-operative delirium in the total hip and knee replacement patient (concurrent), *Journal of Orthopaedic Nursing*, 13(3): 141.

Small, N. and Rhodes, P. (2000) *Too Ill to Talk? User Involvement and Palliative Care*. London: Routledge.

Strathern, D. (1996) Epidural analgesia: educating patients and nurses, *Nursing Standard*, 10(5): 33–66.

Royal College of Anaesthetists, Royal College of Nursing, Association of Anaesthetists of Great Britain and Ireland, British Pain Society and European Society of Regional Anaesthesia and Pain Therapy (2004) *Good Practice in the Management of Continuous Epidural Analgesia in the Hospital Setting*. London: Association of Anaesthetists of Great Britain and Ireland.

Trim, J., Fordyce, F. and Dua, S. (2003) Using clinical governance to standardise an epidural service *Nursing Standard*, 18(9): 43–5.

Welsh Assembly Government (WAG) (2003) *A Strategic Direction for Palliative Care Services in Wales*. Cardiff: Welsh Assembly Government.

Williams, B. and Wheatley, R. (2000) Epidural analgesia for postoperative pain relief, in D.J. Rowbotham (2000) (ed.) *Continuing Medical Education Core Topic*, Bulletin 2, p. 70. Available online at www.rcoa.ac.uk/docs/Bulletin02.pdf (accessed 14 December 2009).

Zwakhalen, S.M., Hamers, J.P., Peijnenburg, R.H. and Berger, M.P. (2007) Nursing staff knowledge and beliefs about pain in elderly nursing home residents with dementia, *Pain Reserve Management*, 12(3): 177–84.

Acute pain management: planning for pain

7

Chapter contents

Introduction
The physical effects of unmanaged acute pain
The surgical stress response
    Cardiovascular effects
    Respiratory effects
    Gastrointestinal effects
Balanced analgesia
Patient-controlled analgesia (PCA)
    What is PCA?
    Basic principles of PCA

Person-centred pain management
    Aims of patient-centred approach
    Ethical considerations
Ensuring adherence to care
The pain management plan
    Problems with setting goals and outcomes
    The plan
    Applying the pain management plan
Summary
Reflective activity
References

Introduction

In Chapter 7 we consider why acute pain needs to be managed and suggest how this can be achieved using a logical and systematic approach. In doing this, we apply some of the principles that we have discussed in previous chapters.

This chapter mainly looks at post-operative pain as a model for acute pain management. While we do this, we should remember that although most post-operative pain, by its very nature, is generally acute and time-limited, it is not the only form of acute pain. One of the major differences between post-operative pain and most other acute pain is that it is **iatrogenic** in nature. That is, caused by the actions of health care professionals, in most cases surgeons, although if we include all **procedural** pains under this category, then any action by health care professionals that produces pain is covered. It should however be borne in mind that the intention is to treat an underlying problem and not to cause pain in itself; in this respect pain after surgery or procedure is an unwelcome side-effect and in our opinion action should always be taken to mitigate it in order to prevent it.

We consider the impact that this unwanted by-product has on patients and address some of the issues that arise while trying to address this. Another difference between post-operative pain and other acute pains is that most acute pain research has focused on this area to the relative neglect of other areas. This means that there is a wealth of information to consider and for this reason we concentrate on the effects of surgical acute pain and planning how to manage it.

This chapter will cover the following seven topics:

1 the physical effects of unmanaged acute pain;
2 the surgical stress response;
3 balanced analgesia;
4 patient-controlled analgesia;
5 person-centred pain management;
6 ensuring adherence to care;
7 the pain management plan.

As a result the following objectives will be addressed:

- identifying the impact of unrelieved acute pain on an individual;
- developing a person-centred approach to pain management;
- producing pain management plans to deal with pain problems.

The physical effects of unmanaged acute pain

Pain relief is desirable not only for humane and moral reasons, but also because adequate pain management maintains and improves physical and psychological welfare (Apfelbaum et al., 2003). Inadequate post-operative analgesia contributes to the development of avoidable complications that may jeopardize recovery (Carr, 2007). Unrelieved pain produces immobility, which leads to muscle loss and weakness and impairs pulmonary function. Lack of movement and reduced tissue oxygenation is a contributing factor to the development of deep vein and pulmonary thromboses (Kehlet and Wilmore, 2002) and increases chest infections and gastric stasis. According to Apfelbaum et al. (2003), other complications that can arise, particularly where there is existing co-morbidity, include coronary ischaemia, myocardial infarction, pneumonia and poor wound healing (see Case study 7.1).

Case study 7.1: acute pain kills

Both Mr Jones, a 53-year-old lecturer and Mrs White a 59-year-old housewife are due to have a thoracic oesophagectomy due to cancer. The anaesthetist visited them pre-operatively and gave them information on post-operative analgesia. Mr Jones having had the risks and benefits explained refused to consent to an epidural in preference for a PCA post-operatively. Following their operations, the patients spent time on the high dependency unit for close observation following major surgery.

The acute pain service visited the patients on their first post-operative day. Mrs White had mild pain only with her epidural whereas Mr Jones had severe pain particularly on deep breathing and coughing despite using his PCA as instructed and having had intravenous paracetamol and rectal diclofenac.

Mr Jones was unable to comply with physiotherapy, could not perform deep breathing or coughing exercises, and consequently developed a chest infection. This progressed to acute respiratory failure requiring assisted ventilation and transfer to the intensive care unit. Fortunately, Mr Jones recovered but stayed in hospital three weeks longer than Mrs White, who had an uneventful recovery.

> **Key point**
>
> Unmanaged acute pain can lead to dangerous complications.

The surgical stress response

The endocrine, metabolic and inflammatory responses to injury and infection result in a variety of physiological changes often grouped together and called the 'surgical stress response' (Kehlet, 1989; Giannoudis et al., 2006). The result of these responses consists of numerous physiological changes promoting **catabolism**, sympathetic activation, **hypercoagulability, immunosupression** and other adverse states in the post-operative patient. The degree of tissue trauma is the main determinant of the extent of the stress response (Giannoudis et al., 2006) but other significant contributors include emotion, pain, nutritional and cardiovascular state. Pain also has an effect on the cardiovascular, respiratory and gastrointestinal systems.

> **Activity 7.1**
>
> In Table 7.1, list some of the effects that acute pain may have on the body's systems.

Cardiovascular effects

Adverse cardiovascular effects exacerbated by pain including tachycardia, hypertension, increased peripheral resistance and cardiac output resulting from the sympathetic overactivity. This increases the work of the myocardium and oxygen consumption which can lead to myocardial ischaemia and infarction (Wu and Liu, 2008), particularly in patients with pre-existing myocardial disease.

Respiratory effects

The respiratory effects of unrelieved pain produce reduced respiratory performance and the ability to cough (Wu and Liu, 2008). This potential problem increases in patients who are elderly, smokers and those with pre-existing respiratory disease (Dunwoody et al., 2008). Respiratory complications are more likely to occur when pain occurs on movement rather than when the patient is resting as dynamic pain interferes with sitting upright, deep breathing and coughing and walking (Kimball et al., 2008). This can result in the patient developing **atelectasis**, chest infections, pneumonia, hypoxia and possible respiratory failure as outlined in Case study 7.1.

Gastrointestinal effects

Pain may slow the normal gut activity after operation, resulting in an increase in the period when intravenous fluids are needed. Inappropriate analgesia may increase the potential for nausea, vomiting and constipation leading to dehydration (Royal College of Surgeons and College of Anaesthetists, 1990). Gastric stasis and even **paralytic ileus** may occur (Dunwoody et al., 2008). However, the precise role of pain on these symptoms is difficult to assess due to the magnitude of other contributing variables such as time spent in pre-operative fasting, the type and duration of anaesthesia and amount of opioid analgesia used.

Cardiovascular system	Respiratory system	Gastrointestinal system

Table 7.1 Effects of acute pain on body systems

Unrelieved pain can directly stimulate production of high levels of catecholamine, the stress hormones, and these modulate immune function, affecting healing and increasing infection risk (Dunwoody et al., 2008). Pain can also indirectly affect catecholamine levels through impeding sleep. This also induces fatigue and emotional distress. These psychological effects of undertreated pain must not be overlooked either given that pain is a biopsychosocial phenomenon. They also include anxiety and fear, anger and aggressiveness and sorrow and depression (Macintyre and Schug, 2007).

Prevention and treatment of post-operative pain can therefore protect the patient against far more than just the unpleasantness of pain (Apfelbaum et al., 2003). If the treatment is effective and promotes early mobilization through eliminating dynamic pain, then it can improve quality of life, reduce adverse clinical events and reduce costs (Kehlet and Wilmore, 2002). This is achievable using combinations of pain management technologies and drugs to produce multimodal or balanced analgesia.

Balanced analgesia

In Chapter 5 we considered the principles behind drug actions and took a broad overview of how different drugs act. It might be useful to review this chapter at this point before considering the concept of balanced or multimodal analgesia. This concept takes advantage of the additive or synergetic effects of combining multiple pain-killing agents whose effect is exerted in different ways. This has been shown to produce more effective analgesia and in some combinations to reduce side-effects as lower doses of opioids can be used (Buvanendran and Kroin, 2009). For example, non-steroidal anti-inflammatory drugs (NSAIDs) and paracetamol seem to have an opioid sparing effect as does the use of regional anaesthetic nerve blocks (Horlocker et al., 2006). Also newer agents such as gabapentin may also produce opioid-reducing benefits (Buvanendran and Kroin, 2009) and delivering well-established drugs in different routes; for example, intravenous paracetamol may also produce better analgesia and reduce opioid consumption (Cattabriga et al., 2007).

Figure 7.1 illustrates the principle of multimodal analgesics. In this you can see that where possible you always use paracetamol first and move up to adding in NSAIDs and opioids with the opioid selected and dose being dependent on the degree of pain assessessed.

Patient-controlled analgesia (PCA)

What is PCA?

In most surgical situations, particularly in elective surgery, we can make broad generalizations about pain. For example, we can plot a general trajectory of pain:

1. intense severe pain for the first day;
2. easing in intensity over the following days as healing occurs;
3. eventually the pain becomes an ache;
4. pain then goes.

Such predictions work on a macroscopic scale, and they are fairly accurate at this level, although differences will occur depending on the type and extent of surgery – a vasectomy will follow a different pain trajectory to a total knee replacement. They can be useful as they tell us what happens over time for the majority of patients and this can give us a 'norm' to which we can compare someone's progress.

While such generalizations have a value, as many cases are lumped together to get these predictions they do not take into account the personal experience of pain. On a personal level these vary considerably from the 'norm' and change with time, activity, level of anxiety, mood and general health. This variability presents a problem in post-operative pain management. It is a reason why relatively inflexible approaches such as bolus opioid intramuscular injections have often failed.

A more flexible approach that rapidly responds to the pain an individual experiences can overcome these problems. One way around this is to adjust the dose of analgesia and administer it rapidly on demand. A practical method of achieving this is through PCA. This gives controlled, small doses of intravenous opioids, at intervals as required. PCA is a:

> *system whereby patients can administer their own intravenous analgesia and titrate the*

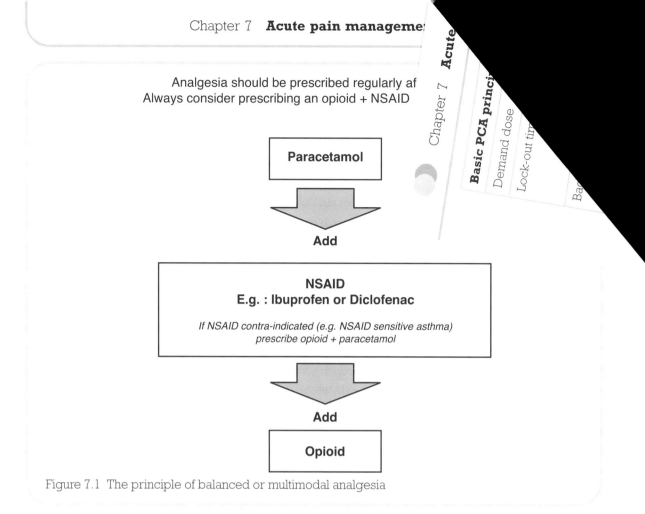

Analgesia should be prescribed regularly af
Always consider prescribing an opioid + NSAID

Paracetamol

Add

NSAID
E.g. : Ibuprofen or Diclofenac

If NSAID contra-indicated (e.g. NSAID sensitive asthma)
prescribe opioid + paracetamol

Add

Opioid

Figure 7.1 The principle of balanced or multimodal analgesia

dose to their own endpoint of pain relief using a small microprocessor controlled pump.

(Charlton, 1997)

PCA is basically a method of self-administration of analgesia. This is something that most people do with over-the-counter medication. If you are at home and you have pain, you may well go to the medicine cupboard and take a painkiller that you had previously bought from a pharmacist or supermarket. Whether or not it is suitable depends on your ability to make an informed decision of when and how much analgesia is needed to treat your pain. This decision is based on your personal preferences and knowledge. Self-administration is therefore a long-established method of managing pain and remains the most usual way to administer analgesia.

In hospital however the situation is different; it involve drugs that are stronger than those the patient will normally come into contact with, they are not familiar with, or due to either legislative or organiza-tional issues, are not responsible for. The trend is to remove personal responsibility for pain relief from the patient by the health care practitioner even though the evidence has demonstrated that they are not necessarily the best at administering analgesia in a manner that is effective for the management of pain. PCA technology provides an opportunity to ensure that patients regain a measure of control over the administration of analgesia to themselves.

The technique for effective pain management using PCA involves making certain that the analgesia is titrated to the patient's pain. To do this you need a method that is easy to use, safe, flexible and fast.

Basic principles of PCA

The strength of PCA is its flexibility (Cashman, 2003). PCA retains the 'on demand' concept of 'as required' intramuscular analgesia while removing the time delays built into this method by organizational constraints. Its basic principle is self-administration. It

129

...ples	
	The amount of drug delivered on each successful press of the PCA button
...e	The minimum interval time between successful doses. The patient can make several demands during this interval but will not receive a dose of the drug
...ckground infusions	A low concentration of the analgesia that is constantly infused. This use is controversial and is mainly restricted to young children
Dose limits	The upper amount of drug a patient can receive in a hour

Table 7.2 Definition of basic PCA principles

does this by manipulating the following: demand dose, lock-out time, background infusions and dose limits (Cashman, 2003) (Table 7.2).

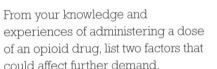

Activity 7.2

From your knowledge and experiences of administering a dose of an opioid drug, list two factors that could affect further demand.

Consider how these two factors can influence the feedback loop described in Fig. 7.2.

PCA is now an established method and usually uses an intravenous infusion device, either a pump or a syringe driver, programmed to deliver a set dose of analgesia when the patient pushes a demand button (Broom and Parsons, 2009). Following this, a predetermined 'lock-out' period allows the patient to continue demanding analgesia as and when they have pain while preventing them from getting too much. In theory this allows for patient variability, through safely topping-up drug plasma levels as the patient experiences pain, in a simple feedback process of pain, demand, relief or further demand until they obtain pain relief (see Fig. 7.2). In reality, several factors 'muddy the water' and we must consider these if we are to have a model that accurately describes the process in real life. Aside from the obvious result that the opioid will remove any pain and therefore no more demand is made, Harmer and MacIntyre (2003) identify three possible factors arising from the side-effects of opioids. These unpleasant adverse effects such as

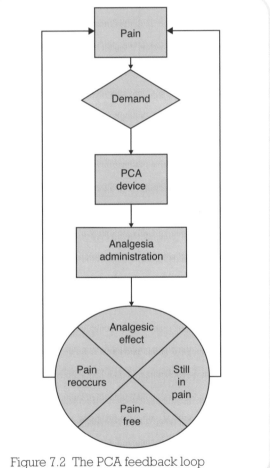

Figure 7.2 The PCA feedback loop

nausea, vomiting, **dysphoria** and sedation, may cause the patient to temper their use of the PCA.

Another definition of PCA is the self-administration of analgesia by methods which consider safety, as well as ability and willingness to exercise control over choice. The increase in autonomy associated with PCA use allows the patient to decide when to administer the next dose. However, as with self-medication at home, a number of influences affect the decision to take another dose; among them are the following four questions:

1. Is the pain still there?
2. Has the analgesia helped?
3. Have I experienced any unpleasant side-effects?
4. Can I take some more analgesia?

Activity 7.3

Think back to the last time you self-administered analgesia for pain relief. How did you respond to these four questions?

1 Is the pain still there?

The answer to this might be a straightforward yes or no; or you might have reduced the severity of the pain but it could still be bothering you. Perhaps the painkillers were not strong enough, they have worn off, or you have exacerbated the pain through activity.

2 Has the analgesia helped?

This might also be a straight yes or no but you might have had some effect but no real benefit in terms of being able to function. For example, the pain decreased a little but not enough for you to feel comfortable, or the pain eased for a short period only and came back long before it was time to have a second dose. A possible explanation is that either the dose was not correct for your needs or the analgesic was not suitable for the severity of your pain.

3 Have I experienced any unpleasant side-effects?

While pain might have been relieved, the analgesia might have produced other problems. If these are very unpleasant, you might have been reluctant to take any further analgesia. The result of this is that you will continue

to have pain. On the other hand, you might have tolerated the side-effects and put up with them as the lesser of two evils. Your decision balances the severity of the side-effect and the risks you associate with them against pain severity. This can be a very difficult decision and has consequences for pain management.

4 Can I take some more analgesia?

In PCA this is regulated by the lock-out period. Prescriptions carry recommended intervals for repeating doses; however, when self-administering over-the-counter analgesia such as paracetamol there is no physical barrier to taking an overdose as there is in a PCA device.

Other considerations also affect decisions about pain management, which include:

- previous experiences of the analgesia and the route used;
- vicarious experiences, such as stories from relatives;
- a reluctance to take drugs and a desire to 'tough it out';
- fear of strong analgesics;
- the mitigating effect of drugs that prevent or reduce side-effects, such as anti-emetics and attitudes of others.

Some ways of resolving these issues were covered in Chapter 6 when we discussed education and information-giving. Another important aspect is to consider what it means to be person-centred in your approach to managing pain.

Person-centred pain management

Adopting a patient-centred approach to health care has the benefit of addressing these issues as patient involvement is integral. Stewart et al. (1995) describe a method for producing a patient-centred approach to care. This has six integrated components:

1. exploring and interpreting both the disease and the illness experience;
2. understanding the whole person and acknowledging that the patient

a) is more than his or her symptoms
b) has ideas, concerns, and expectations
c) may have other problems that need attention and,
d) often has continuing problems

3 finding common ground with the patient about the problem and its management;
4 incorporating prevention and health promotion;
5 enhancing the carer-patient relationship;
6 being realistic about time and resources.

In this model an awareness of these criteria will enable health carers to be in a better position to bring about outcomes that the patient wants and enable patients to take responsibility for their own health and to make judicious use of health services.

Person-centred pain management can be considered to be a way of providing care that provides patients with the means to exert choice and influence their pain management plan. This can be viewed as an extension of PCA. The key factors in ensuring you provide care in this way are:

■ effective communication;
■ information-giving, so that a knowledgeable decision can be made about the best method to manage their pain;

■ promotion of patient autonomy, allowing the patient or client to make decisions about their care and respecting their decision;
■ advocacy – or supporting the patient in the decision-making process;
■ non-maleficence – acting in the best interests of the patients, ensuring that both their decisions and your subsequent actions based on those decisions do no harm to the patient.

> **Key point**
>
> Person-centred pain management ensures the patient is integral to the process of managing their pain.

Aims of patient-centred approach

The main aims of a patient-centred approach are to reduce patients' concerns as far as possible and to give clear explanations so patients can understand and remember in order to ensure their commitment to the planned pain management (Fuertes et al., 2007).

This might seem like an easy and straightforward recipe to follow but in reality these principles may and quite often do interfere with each other. Consider the following Case study 7.2.

Case study 7.2

Henry James is aged 76 and until six weeks ago was a heavy smoker; he hasn't smoked since being advised by the surgeon to stop. He finds breathing difficult and suffers with chronic obstructive pulmonary disease. He suffers from peripheral vascular disease and he has a history of chronic foot ulcers that have not healed and have become infected and necrotic. He is going to theatre to have a femoral artery graft in an attempt to improve the circulation to his feet and hopefully help his feet heal. Because he was such a heavy smoker and has a bad chest the anaesthetist is very reluctant to give him a general anaesthetic and Mr James has agreed to have epidural anaesthesia.

Mr James was taking anticoagulant therapy but this has been reduced and he is currently on a low molecular weight heparin injection once a day. Despite suffering from peripheral vascular disease he has normal kidney function.

When the acute pain team visits Mr James prior to surgery to discuss his post-operative pain relief, they find he is not anxious about the epidural as his daughter had one for a caesarean section and it worked very well.

A range of options for managing his pain are discussed with Mr James and because he will have an epidural inserted for his anaesthetic, it is decided to continue with this for his post-operative analgesia.

Ethical considerations

In this case there is a conflict as epidurals are usually contraindicated when a patient is on anti-coagulant therapy. However, Mr James's health is so poor that there is little choice but to perform an epidural anaesthetic. The conflict here is between what is best for the patient and the risks that this has for his recovery. Where such conflicts exist, a person-centred approach can be ensured by adopting the following two actions:

1. devolvement of decision-making to the patient;
2. developing the patient's understanding of his health.

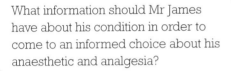

Activity 7.4

What information should Mr James have about his condition in order to come to an informed choice about his anaesthetic and analgesia?

The first thing that needs to be considered is that Mr James is a high-risk candidate for surgery. If we look at Table 7.3 we can see that his ASA (American Society of Anesthesiology) score for anaesthetic risk is at least III and is possibly as high as IV. Although this is not a perfect method of assessing risk (Walker,

2002), it does provide an indication of how serious Mr James's risk of surgery is and explains the reluctance of the anaesthetist to administer a general anaesthetic.

As there is a significant risk that Mr James would have been greatly harmed by a general anaesthetic, he should have been informed of this risk and other options explored. As there is a need to perform surgery in order to attempt to cure his underlying condition and heal his wounds, the most reasonable alternative is an epidural anaesthetic. However, as we discussed in Chapter 6, every procedure has risks as well as benefits. We examine those that are specific to Mr James.

The first and possibly most significant of these risks is that Mr James is taking anticoagulants. MacIntyre et al. (2003) identify the concurrent use of anticoagulant drugs including warfarin and heparin as major risk factors in the development of epidural haematomas. Normally these are very rare events although they have potentially devastating consequences. Mintzer et al. (2002) state that they are so rare that there is no good evidence on their incidence to provide information about their cause or prevention and that case history and anecdote are the main method used for reporting them. There is little or no statistical probability associated with them, although Rathmell et al. (2003) cite one source as stating a risk of 0.0007 per cent.

This is a potential dilemma, as epidurals pose

Class	Physical status	Example
I	A completely healthy patient	A fit patient with an inguinal hernia
II	A patient with mild systemic disease	Essential hypertension, mild diabetes without end organ damage
III	A patient with severe systemic disease that is not incapacitating	Angina, moderate to severe COPD
IV	A patient with incapacitating disease that is a constant threat to life	Advanced COPD, cardiac failure
V	A moribund patient who is not expected to live 24 hours with or without surgery	Ruptured aortic aneurysm, massive pulmonary embolism
E	Emergency case	

Table 7.3 ASA score
Source: Walker (2002)

a hypothetical risk of haematoma, but the risk is very small and in practical terms is unquantifiable because of the lack of good data (Federal Drug Agency, 2002). However, anticoagulants greatly increase the risk, although we cannot quantify this. In the past standard practice in the USA was to use a higher dose than in the UK and Europe and this coupled with higher epidural usage might have led to a greater incidence.

Mr James does not take NSAIDs and has good renal function and is on a reduced dose of low molecular weight heparin. Should he be informed of this risk because he has no choice about having an epidural anaesthetic if he is going to have surgery?

When considering this dilemma the risks need to be balanced against the benefits. First, the risk of not having the operation against having the operation has been put to Mr James and he has opted for having the operation. The consequences of not proceeding are severe chronic pain, malnutrition, loss of mobility, infectious gangrene, need for a amputation, septicaemia and death. Second, the risks of an epidural versus a general anaesthetic have been considered and because of his ASA grade the risk of morbidity or death from a general anaesthetic are more likely than the risk of an epidural haematoma.

However, while Mr James will be having an epidural for his anaesthetic and because of the likely length of the operation this will probably involve the placement of a catheter, is there a risk that maintaining the epidural infusion past the anaesthetic to provide analgesia increases the risk of a haematoma? We can find no evidence that the duration of an indwelling catheter contributes or does not contribute to the incidence of haematoma. It seems likely that the event that is going to cause a haematoma is the insertion of the needle and the threading of the catheter. There is possibly a risk of bleeding when the catheter is removed as any clots that have formed might be disturbed, or trauma may occur to blood vessels in the epidural space.

In our opinion, as the risky process of insertion will take place, there seems to be no evidence that harm will occur through continued use of the inserted epidural catheter for pain relief. It seems then reasonable to inform Mr James about the risk of an epidural *per se* with regard to haematomas but not to suggest that this risk is prolonged by the duration of analgesia.

The decisions we take about the information we give to patients is ultimately a moral decision. Most of the time these are quite easy ones to make; in Mr James's case however they are quite difficult. We have considered this question in terms of our clinical experience and through writing this chapter. It might be that you differ in your opinion. The important thing is that you keep the patient in mind when weighing up these decisions and you have followed logical reasoning based on the best available evidence.

However, even when you have been logical in your reasoning and you produce a pain management treatment based on the patient's prior beliefs and knowledge, it is important to recognize that this knowledge is imperfect and can always be improved on. Adapting the plan in the light of new knowledge can help you manage the patient and his pain realistically. One of the reasons for doing this is to ensure compliance or adherence to care.

>
> **Key point**
>
> There are many reasons why individuals do not adhere to a pain management plan. Understanding these reasons will enable more effective pain management.

Ensuring adherence to care

Compliance with treatment and care is an important but often neglected area of pain management. Compliance with medication is problematic and, because pain has been believed to be a motivator to take analgesia, there exists a prevailing view that patients are likely to 'abuse' medication by overusing analgesia. However, when this premise is examined this is clearly not the case. One study (Heavner et al., 1996) demonstrated that patients taking paracetamol for pain failed to achieve therapeutic plasma paracetamol levels in a range of commonly prescribed co-analgesics, despite being advised to take their analgesia regularly. A more recent study, Garbez et al. (2006), established a significant non-adherence rate to analgesia, including non-collection of prescriptions among emergency room patients. As both studies involve patients with ongoing pain, it is difficult to believe that they would 'forget' to take their medication – a factor that is put forward as a reason for non-compliance in drug-taking for other conditions. We therefore need to consider what other reasons might exist for that influence compliance.

There are many reasons why a patient or client might not comply with their pain management. For example:

- It may not suit the patient's lifestyle.
- It is too complicated for the patient to bother to follow.
- The advice is related to a diagnosis that the patient is trying hard to reject.
- It does not fit in with the patient's own view of the problem.
- There is a lack of emotional support from those around them.

Some other reasons may include a lack of time or resources to support the patient. Additionally, it should be remembered that inpatients are very reluctant to be active in their acute pain care and commonly act as passive recipients of care (Manias et al., 2006); this puts a greater burden on care providers to ensure that communication is effective and care is shared appropriately.

Arkes (2003) prefers to refer to non-compliance as a form of 'patient decision-making'. After all they have made a decision not to follow the advice and treatment given to them. This perspective implies that patients have reasons for not taking analgesia that need to be valued. It also moves us away from a paternalistic approach, where our language implies that we consider the patient or client to be a child. Some of these reasons include:

- *The patient has to choose between conflicting symptoms* For example, between pain relief and drug-induced nausea or sedation. Of course by now you should be thinking 'those symptoms are likely to occur because of poor management'. However, we need to realize that we are discussing what the patient believes their choice is.

  This leads a person to consider how much pain they are willing to tolerate before they will 'take something for it'. If this means that the pain interferes with their daily life – for example, they do not get out of bed – then we may feel we are entering serious ethical grounds as the patient is not

acting in their own best interests. Of course, they may not know the consequences of not following the treatment and we therefore have to decide whether or not we should tell them these.

- *Omission bias* Knowing the risks of non-compliance does not always produce compliance. Omission bias can occur even when the patient considers the risks of not acting to be greater than having the treatment because they would feel responsible for the consequences of any action but would not feel responsible if something just happened as a natural effect of not complying with care.

  This is a particular issue where carers make decisions about dependants' health. A classic example is seen in decision-making about the use of opioids in terminal illness that may also be affected by this if a carer believes that their involvement in a decision to administer higher doses of opioid will hasten death.

- *Discount rates* If a patient has a choice between two therapies; one that offers a small gain immediately and another that offers a bigger gain in the future their decision will depend on the following factors:

- How easy the treatments are in terms of commitment;
- How much bigger the gain is from the delayed treatment.

If a person has a choice between an immediate benefit and a longer benefit, they are only likely to wait if they are convinced that it will be better for them to do so. If both treatments require significant effort, then the quicker therapy becomes even more attractive even if it involves more pain and suffering in the short term. This may explain why patients prefer spinal surgery to a back pain management programme.

Discounting is the main reason why patients make an immediate decision to undergo a therapy and then fail to reattend and continue with it. They will initially agree if the treatment is immediately available but by the time their next appointment comes along sufficient time has passed to allow them to rethink the degree of benefit they will receive.

Discounting works in reverse as well. Women who previously wanted a natural childbirth are more likely to agree to intrusive pain relief if it is offered while they are in labour.

- *Framing* If the risk of not adhering to a pain management plan is discussed at the time of giving information, people are more likely to respond favourably to a therapy. According to Arkes (2003) this is because the information is framed in terms of losses and people are reluctant to lose something they already have. This applies particularly well to situations where there is likely to be a deterioration in the status quo. So if adherence to taking analgesia post-operatively is couched in terms of prevention of identified complications it is more likely to be successful.
- *Assessing probabilities* This can be a source of conflict between health carers and patients whether they decide to comply or not. According to Arkes (2003), people are more likely to be optimistic about outcomes than health professionals. If a person decides to comply with a treatment they are likely to believe that they will get the maximum gain from this treatment and avoid the side-effects. If, as is often the case, they do not then they can believe they have been misinformed by their health carers. Conversely, where a person decides that they will not adhere to a therapy, they are more likely to believe they will escape the consequences of non-adherence.
- *Predicting utility* An accurate assessment of the likelihood of an outcome occurring is essential for good decision-making. This can be relatively easy to achieve in an acute pain situation, where as in chronic pain or palliative situations, it is often difficult to predict what their health state would be like if they were to undergo a treatment. Even when there is adequate information often they make an assumption that their life will be instantly and significantly improved when often the best that they can hope for is a slight improvement. This can lead to non-adherence.

> **Key point**
>
> Using a problem-solving approach as documented in a care plan can be an effective way of planning patient-centred care.

The pain management plan

Problems with setting goals and outcomes

Some of the problems may arise because the patient is unaware of the goals of the team, resources available and current evidence influencing pain management decision. Therefore, they are relying on their own beliefs. This makes them very vulnerable. They are a patient in pain against a team of professionals. The pressure on the patient to conform to the wishes of the team will be high and if they do not conform, they run the risk of being labelled as a difficult patient with possible consequences that their ongoing and future care will be jeopardized.

Alternatively, they may feel strongly that they are aware of the goals of the team and the resources available as well as the evidence. They may therefore feel that they are not being offered the most appropriate treatment for them. This may be because:

- the treatment option is not working for them; that is, they have tried it and are still in pain;
- they have had a poor experience with the offered method previously;
- they may have researched or investigated the area of pain and pain management and may feel they are more knowledgeable than the practitioner. This may be particularly true in chronic pain and palliative care where patients are 'experts' in their condition and the conveniences of modern technology mean they can access up-to-date research in the area. This may be in contrast to busy health professionals who may be generalists with a particular interest in a different field of health;
- they may have strong feelings about Western health care and express a desire to seek more holistic complementary ways of managing their pain.

Health carers have a duty to care for someone which means they must consider what the patient understands about the treatment that has been offered to them and must bear this in mind when helping them to understand their options. They may need more information or education to do this. As we have seen there may be a discrepancy between what the patient expects and the outcome that a health professional expects.

Problem	Goal	Plan	Evaluation
Pain after surgery	To be pain free	1. Patient's pain to be assessed regularly 2. If patient is in pain analgesia is to be given as prescribed 3. Effect of analgesia is to be recorded in the nursing notes 4. If patient is still in pain after analgesia is given then the doctor should be informed 5. Comfort measures to be used as appropriate.	Patient was in pain

Table 7.4 A poorly designed care plan

A nursing care plan is a good example of a professionally led outcome indicator. Ideally, a problem is identified and then a goal is determined against which a plan can be drawn up and progress can be measured through evaluation. We need to be logical and evidence-based; however, this is not always the case. Table 7.4 is an example of a nursing care plan that we have regularly seen in practice in a surgical setting.

Activity 7.5

Consider the care plan in Table 7.4. Can you spot any problems with it?

The problem with this care plan is that the stated outcome or goal is quite definite but is unrealistic. To say that 'to be pain free' is an aspiration but it is not a clinical possibility. You only have to have one patient to tell you they are in pain for it to fail as an outcome and if you were to use this as a measure of how efficient you are at delivering pain management, you would be inviting unnecessary criticism. Indeed the very term 'pain management' implies that someone must have pain in order for you to be able to manage it.

The danger of using such a statement is that it might either raise the expectations of your ability to deal with pain beyond the competence of your ability to deliver care. Or it might reinforce a patient's opinion that you have no idea about their pain.

It is more appropriate to write this goal in a way that can be used to accurately measure the quality of care. To achieve this you need to do the following:

1. have a reasonable idea of what the patient can expect for pain after surgery;
2. individualize the care by involving the patient in decisions;
3. alongside the patient decide on what a reasonable course of action is;
4. focus on the management of pain.

A goal that achieves this will acknowledge that pain can occur but that there are interventions that should work for this pain. We would consider a reasonable goal to contain a statement that the patient's 'pain will be managed'. How this will be achieved would then be detailed in the treatment plan and the evaluation would then focus on how effective the pain management was. This would allow you to adjust care according to the patient's preferences.

To set goals in a patient-centred way, there are a few rules that need to be followed:

- *Be specific* Avoid woolly and vague goals and focus on clearly defined goals that have clear criteria. We advocate basing the goal on a pain assessment score and setting a time limit. For example, using a VAS where 0 = 'no pain' and 10 = 'worst pain imaginable', a goal could be that 'patients will *experience a pain score of no more than 3*, one hour after taking oral analgesia, during the first 48 hours after surgery'.

- *Be reasonable* Either set small and moderate goals or if setting large goals, then identify the stages you would need to go through to get there and break the goal down into these small achievable steps. In the example above we set a score of 3, one hour after taking oral analgesia as a reasonable outcome for someone in the first 48 hours after surgery because we acknowledge that it can be very difficult to reduce pain below this without increasing other risks. Also a score of 3 represents a degree of mild pain where someone can function and act to reduce complications of surgery. This might however require some explanation to the patient.
- *Focus on needs* A patient-centred approach means that patients should be asked about what they want and not what you as a health professional can give them. If they want something you haven't got or haven't offered them, then you are going to fail to meet their outcome. If you are going to use a specific pain assessment tool, you need to make sure they understand what it means and that they agree with your goal. In the example given under the point above 'be specific'; it is no use stating that an acceptable pain score is 3 if they want the score to be 1.

The other problem with the care plan in Table 7.4 is that it lacks internal consistency. The goal states that the patient will be pain-free but the plan then details how to manage pain. The evaluation clearly identifies the patients as having pain and therefore the goal needs to be changed. The evaluation also focuses on the presence or absence of pain only and not on the treatment plan.

The plan

The care plan in Table 7.4 also lacks specific statements in the plan. There are not many concrete items that care can be measured against and those that do exist are process-oriented rather than patient-oriented. For example, you could measure whether the effect of analgesia was recorded in the notes but how does this help the person if the analgesia is ineffective? In other words, this is not a very relevant outcome to use for this problem.

We would advocate that a pain management plan considers the following:

- an evaluation of existing pain;
- a regime to reduce or eliminate the pain;
- a description of which actions to take including analgesic modalities and the use of appropriate non-pharmacological measures;
- an evaluation of the intervention, what to do if actions do not work or problems occur.

An evaluation of the pain

The plan should incorporate an appropriate assessment of the pain which records its intensity, location and cause. This should be quantifiable, measured and recorded. It should also be ongoing throughout the course of the pain and should be used to identify discrepancies between what is predicted to occur and what actually occurs. The assessment should be consistent and whenever possible the patient should be taught how to perform the assessment themselves.

To achieve this we would advocate naming a particular assessment tool in the plan and making sure the patient understands and can use this tool. We would also expect patients to be encouraged to self-report their pain using this tool. In order to do this your care plan should include educating patients in the pain assessment tool.

The assessment should also realistically evaluate the pain therapy. This should take place both before and after the intervention and needs to be mindful of the nature of the intervention. For example, the route and dose of a drug must be considered. It would be worthless to evaluate oral analgesia before it has time to take effect, but if the same time scale is used for intravenous analgesia, then any benefit is likely to have passed and the patient would be in pain again.

Evaluation should also consider the clinical situation. We have seen that good post-operative pain management will reduce complications as patients will be able to move and help themselves. Treatments need to be evaluated on the basis of ability to function. If a patient is only assessed when resting, then you have not tested the efficacy of your care against actions like deep breathing or mobilizing, and this leaves them vulnerable to developing complications.

Description of what action to take

Again these should be specific and relate to local guidelines and protocols. They should record how effective the treatments are and any action that is taken to make them more effective. They should also describe action to take in the event of any adverse events. Additionally, they should bear in mind the specific treatment. If it is a drug the mode and route of delivery needs to be considered. For example, where intravenous opioids are used in a PCA, they should identify the potential problem of respiratory depression and detail what action to take to rectify this.

What to do if actions do not work

A good pain management plan should also detail what action to take when an existing plan fails. This should include information such as who to refer to if changes are needed and how to document these changes. For example, if a painkiller has been administered and has no effect, then the person responsible for changing the prescription should be identified in the plan. When a change is required this should be recorded along with the action taken and the pain management plan amended to reflect this.

Applying the pain management plan

We have been considering pain management in terms of acute post-operative pain but these principles that we have highlighted can be transferred to the management of any acute pain situation; for example, acute cardiac pain, sickle cell pain or multiple rib fractures, as seen in a flail chest. We have also used nursing care plans as an example of how to do this. You may not use these in your area of practice; perhaps you use integrated care pathways. This does not matter as long as the pain has a management plan in place that is principled and logical. The following activity will ask you to consider some of these principles in a patient in your care.

Activity 7.6

Review an existing acute pain care plan using the criteria outlined in Table 7.5.

Activity 7.7

Having reviewed this care plan, consider how you would adjust it in order to produce a person-centred pain management plan.

Summary

In this chapter we have considered acute pain through the lens of the post-operative experience. This has been done for reasons of expediency as there are so many acute pains and we have a limited space to consider them. Instead of delving into the detail of each type of acute pain, we have endeavoured to provide a structure that considers what the main problems with acute pain are and evaluates how you can logically tackle all acute pains using a structured pain management. The aim of this has been to put the person in pain at the centre of the action. In doing this we wished to communicate the following ideas:

- Acute pain may have a trajectory that diminishes over time but this is not an excuse not to act to reduce it.
- Unrelieved, severe acute pain has life-threatening consequences.
- A disciplined and structured approach can resolve acute pain.
- Such an approach will only work if the person in pain is actively involved in planning their care.

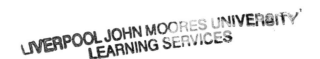

Principle	Criteria	Your assessment
Person-centredness	Is the patient involvement in the plan of care, e.g. choice of treatment? Is there evidence of improving understanding? Do goals relate to the patient's needs at that time?	
Communication	How aware is the patient of the content of the care plan? Have they been informed of how they can help themselves? For example, do they use the pain assessment tool? Have they been told when to inform carers about their pain? Is there evidence of patient education? Are all carers using the care plan? Are actions and variations in care documented? Is there a record of evaluation?	
Safety	Is the plan specific to the treatment choice? For example, does timing of assessment relate to mode and type of analgesia? Does the plan refer to local guidelines and policies? Are side-effects and adverse events monitored and is specific action detailed?	
Efficacy	Does evaluation relate to ability to function? Does the plan specify timescales and specific actions to take? Does the plan adequately address complications and side-effects, e.g. nausea? Is there evidence of a plan review and update? Does the plan change over to time to reflect changing patient needs?	

Table 7.5 Criteria for writing a care plan

Reflective activity

As a conclusion to this chapter consider how using a systematic approach to acute pain management could improve your practice. Try to be detailed in your reflection and follow the guidelines below:

- *State* which elements of the chapter will help you in your future practice and consider what areas need further study. For example, do you need to learn more about different methods of analgesia?
- *Elaborate:* be specific in terms of how this knowledge and understanding can be used in practice. For example, how can you make the care you deliver more person-centred?

- *Give examples:* of specific areas of practice which should be reviewed. For example, do you evaluate your care and, if you do, do you use a care plan or some other systematic method of organizing care, such as an integrated care pathway (ICP)? How person-centred are the care plans or ICPs you are using? Are individual care plans used or do you use a generic one? It is worth bearing in mind that the use of a generic care plan is not necessarily a bad idea as long as it is carefully constructed.

What are the *implications* if acute pain management is not person-centred?

You may prefer to use a reflective model such as Gibbs's (1988) to guide your reflection (see Appendix at the end of this book). Think of a specific example as the starting point; for example, an incident where patient-centred care did not occur. When analysing the situation draw on this chapter's theory to support your discussion and demonstrate your understanding. As a result your reflection should examine the key principles that:

- a disciplined and structured approach can resolve acute pain;
- such an approach will only work if the person in pain is actively involved in planning their care.

References

Apfelbaum, J.L., Chen, C., Mehta, S.S. and Gan, T.J. (2003) Postoperative pain experience: results from a national survey suggest postoperative pain continues to be undermanaged, *Anesthsia and Analgesia*, 97(2), 534–40.

Arkes, H.R. (2003) The psychology of patient decision making in M.B. Max and J. Lynn (eds) *Symptom Research: Methods and Opportunities*. Available online at www.symptomresearch.nih.gov/chapter_4/chaauthorbio.htm (accessed 21 June 2010).

Broom, M. and Parsons, G. (2009) Patient-controlled analgesia, in A. Glasper, G. McEwing, and J. Richardson (eds) *Foundation Skills for Caring Using Student-centred Learning* (pp. 310–17) London: Palgrave Macmillan.

Buvanendran, A. and Kroin, K.S. (2009): Multimodal analgesia for controlling acute postoperative pain, *Acute Pain*, 11(3–4): 145–6.

Carr, E. (2007) Barriers to effective pain management, *Journal of Perioperative Practice*, 17(5): 200.

Cashman, J. (2003) Routes of administration, in D.J. Rowbotham and P.E. MacIntyre (ed.) *Clinical Pain Management: Acute Pain* (Chapter 10). London: Arnold.

Cattabriga, I., Pacini, D., Lamazza, G., Talarico, F., Di Bartolomeo, R., Grillone, G. et al. (2007) Intravenous paracetamol as adjunctive treatment for postoperative pain after cardiac surgery: a double blind randomized controlled trial, *European Journal of Cardio-thoracic Surgery*, 32(3): 527–31.

Charlton, E. (1997) *The Management of Postoperative Pain Practical Procedures, Anaesthesia Update*, 2(1–7). Available online at www.nda.ox.ac.uk/wfsa/html/u07/u07_003.htm (accessed 28 August 2009).

Dunwoody, C.J., Krenzischek, D.A., Pasero, C., Rathmell, J.P. and Polomano, R.C. (2008) Assessment, physiological monitoring, and consequences of inadequately treated acute pain, *Pain Management Nursing*, 9(1) (Supplement 1), 11–21.

Federal Drug Agency (2002) *Spinal and Epidural Hematomas: Low Molecular Weight Heparin Drug Labels*. Available online at www.fda.gov/medwatch/SAFETY/2002/lovenox_PI.pdf (accessed November 2004).

Fuertes, J.N., Mislowack, A., Bennett, J., Paul, L., Gilbert, T.C., Fontan, G. et al. (2007) The physician-patient working alliance, *Patient Education and Counselling*, 66(1), 29–36.

Garbez, R.O., Chan, G.K., Neighbor, M. and Puntillo, K. (2006) Pain after discharge: a pilot study of factors associated with pain management and functional status, *Journal of Emergency Nursing*, 32(4): 288–93.

Giannoudis, P.V., Dinopoulos, H., Chalidis, B. and Hall, G.M. (2006) Surgical stress response, *Injury*, 37 (Supplement 5): S3–S9.

Gibbs, G. (1988) *Learning by Doing: A Guide & Teaching and Learning Methods*. Oxford: Further Education Unit, Oxford Polytechnic.

Harmer, M. and MacIntyre, P.E. (2003) Patient controlled analgesia in D.J. Rowbotham and P.E. MacIntyre (2003) (eds) *Clinical Pain Management: Acute Pain* (Chapter 11) London: Arnold.

Heavner, J.E., Shi, B., Diede, J. and Racz, G. (1996). Acetaminophen (paracetamol) use and blood concentration in pain patients, *Pain Digest*, 6: 215–18.

Horlocker, T.T., Kopp, S.L., Pagnano, M.W. and Hebl, J.R. (2006) Analgesia for total hip and knee arthroplasty: a multimodal pathway featuring peripheral nerve block, *Journal of the American Academy of Orthopaedic Surgeons*, 14(3): 126–35.

Kehlet, H. (1989) Surgical stress: the role of pain and analgesia, *British Journal of Anaesthesia*, 63(2), 189–195.

Kehlet, H. and Wilmore, D.W. (2002) Multimodal strategies to improve surgical outcome, *The American Journal of Surgery*, 183: 630–41.

Kimball, W.R., Carwood, C.M., Chang, Y., McKenna, J.M., Peters, L.E. and Ballantyne, J.C. (2008) Effect of effort pain after upper abdominal surgery on two independent measures of respiratory function, *Journal of Clinical Anesthesia*, 20(3): 200–5.

Macintyre, P.E. and Schug, S.A. (2007) *Acute Pain Management: A Practical Guide*. Philadelphia, PA: Elsevier Saunders.

MacIntyre, P.E., Upton, R.N. and Ludbrook, G.L. (2003) Acute pain management in the elderly patient, in D.J. Rowbotham and P.E. MacIntyre (eds) *Clinical Pain Management: Acute Pain* (pp. 463–83). London: Arnold.

Manias, E., Botti, M. and Bucknall, T. (2006). Patients' decision-making strategies for managing postoperative pain, *The Journal of Pain*, 7(6): 428–37.

Minzter, B.H., Johnson, R.F. and Grimm, B.J. (2002) The practice of thoracic epidural analgesia: a survey of academic medical centers in the United States, *Anesthesia and Analgesia*, 95: 472–5.

Rathmel, J.P., Neal, J.M. and Liu, S.S. (2003) Outcome Measurements in Acute Pain Management, in D.J. Rowbotham and P.E. MacIntyre (eds) *Clinical Pain Management: Acute Pain* (Chapter 8) London: Arnold.

Royal College of Surgeons of England and the College of Anaesthetists (1990) *Report of the Working Party on Pain After Surgery*, London.

Stewart, M., Brown, J.B., Weston, W.W., McWhinney, I.R., McWilliam, C.L. and Freeman, T.R. (1995) *Patient-centred Medicine Transforming the Clinical Method*. Thousand Oaks, CA: Sage Publications.

Walker, R. (2002) *ASA and CEPOD Scoring Anaesthesia*, 14(5): 1. Available online at www.nda.ox.ac.uk/wfsa/html/u14/u1405_01.htm (accessed September 2004).

Wu, C.L. and Liu, S.S. (2008) Outcomes, efficacy, and complications from acute postoperative pain management, in M.D. Honorio, M.D. Benzon, P. James et al. (eds) *Raj's Practical Management of Pain*, 4th edn. (pp. 1219–233). Philadelphia, PA: Mosby.

Chronic pain management

8

Chapter contents

Introduction
The problem of chronic pain
The prevalence of chronic pain in the UK and Europe
  Location of pain
  The economic effects of chronic pain
Chronic pain and chronic pain syndrome (CPS)
  Adapting to chronic pain
  Maladapting to chronic pain
  Depression

Specific treatment approaches
  Reducing the risk of developing chronic pain
The chronic pain management plan
  Patients' perceptions
Dealing with pain behaviours
  Combating fear avoidance strategies
  Activity cycling
  Dealing with anxiety, depression and anger
Summary
Reflective activity
References

Introduction

Chronic pain is widespread and for many sufferers is a largely unresolved health care problem. It limits the potential well-being of sufferers causing both psychosocial and physical problems. Many conventional pain therapies and management techniques are either ineffective or have a partial or short duration of action. This forces people with chronic pain to seek help or to demand repeat treatments and this can promote dependency. This coupled with the deleterious effect of constant or continuous pain creates a disability mindset. The evidence base suggests that approaches that address issues such as independence and quality of life are effective for those people with chronic pain who do not respond to conventional treatments or for whom conventional treatments are no longer an option.

Chronic pain affects approximately one in five Europeans (Breivik et al., 2006) and it is estimated that this incidence will increase as the population ages (IASP/EFIC 2004–2005a, b; IASP, 2006–2007), and as a result of diseases such as diabetes (Jensen et al., 2006) and stroke becoming more prevalent. Only 1–2 per cent of chronic pain is caused by cancer and it is thought that policy makers have overlooked the important health problem of chronic pain caused by non-malignant disease (IASP/EFIC, 2004–2005b).

In Chapter 1 we offered a definition of chronic pain and in Chapter 4 the assessment of chronic pain. We do not intend to repeat that content here other than through a brief reference to key points and therefore you may wish to revise that content before proceeding with this chapter.

There are five broad areas that will be covered in this chapter they are:

① the prevalence of chronic pain in the UK and Europe;
② chronic pain and chronic pain syndromes (CPS);
③ specific treatment approaches;
④ the chronic pain management plan;
⑤ dealing with pain behaviours.

As a result the following objectives will be achieved:

- to identify the extent of chronic pain;
- to consider what the chronic pain experience involves;
- to differentiate between chronic pain and CPS;
- to consider approaches that can help people with CPS.

The problem of chronic pain

Chronic pain is an unpleasant sensory and emotional experience associated with actual or potential tissue damage that persists beyond the expected time frame for healing or that occurs in disease processes in which healing may never occur (IASP, 1986).

Chronic pain differs from acute pains in terms of its duration, identifiable cause and uncertainty about its end point. It has become customary to define a pain experience as being chronic if it has lasted for six months or more although some authorities suggest that three months should be the defining point. There are three aspects of chronic pain that are frequently problematic and prove frustrating for individuals:

① the lack of diagnosis in terms of its actual cause, although this is not always the case as many sufferers attributed the pain to a specific diagnosis. This can prove a difficult barrier for both individual and professional and can be a source of psychological trauma;
② the unpredictable nature of the pain's end point. Without a foreseeable end to the experience individuals can lose hope and succumb to this persistent stressor;
③ the attitude and beliefs generally held about chronic pain and the sort of person who suffers from chronic pain by those around them.

The prevalence of chronic pain in the UK and Europe

In many studies the focus has been on the prevalence of chronic pain in specific diseases. For example Parsons et al. (2005) conducted a survey involving 4,100 primary care patients and identified a prevalence rate for chronic musculoskeletal pain of 47 per cent.

The prevalence of chronic pain in the general population is less but still very significant. A survey of chronic pain in Europe (Breivik et al., 2006) demonstrated a 19 per cent prevalence (sample of 46 394) of pain for six months or longer. This is higher than the estimation of 11 per cent in the USA (Hardt et al.'s., 2008) and 11.8 per cent in Canada (Ospini and Harstall's (2002). All these studies suggest a lower rate than the World Health Organization (WHO) findings of 20–30 per cent from 1998 (Gureje, 1998), although these differences may be explained in part by differing assessment criteria.

The Breivik et al. (2006: 289) survey offered comprehensive data on the nature of the chronic pain experience. They were particularly clear about the definition used when indicating their 19 per cent prevalence:

moderate or severe pain of at least six months duration, had experienced pain in the last month, experienced pain at least two times per week. They rated their pain intensity when they last experienced pain at least 5 on a 10-point NRS (numerical rating scale)

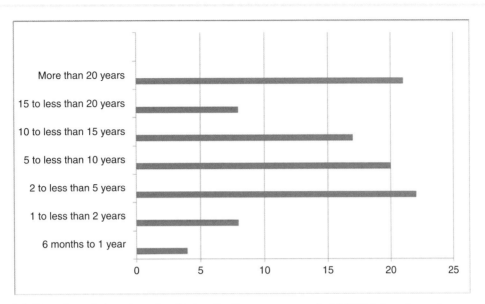

Figure 8.1 Duration of chronic pain of intensity 5 or more on a 1–10 NRS intensity scale
Source: Breivik et al. (2006)

between 1 = no pain and 10 = the worst pain imaginable.

The prevalence varied between countries with the highest in Norway (30 per cent) and the lowest in Spain (12 per cent). They also noted some within country differences. Women (56 per cent) were more likely to suffer with chronic pain as were people within the 41–60 age groups. Their findings also illustrated the prolonged nature of the suffering of these individuals with 21 per cent of the respondents reporting the duration of the pain as being 20 years or more (Fig. 8.1).

Location of pain

The lower back is identified as the most frequent single site of chronic pain with a prevalence of 23 per cent (Parsons et al., 2005) and 18 per cent (Breivik et al., 2006), respectively, for the cited authors; although Breivik et al.'s survey also identified a 24 per cent prevalence for back pain that did not specify a specific site. Table 8.1 shows the most common chronic pain by site in descending order of prevalence.

Breivik et al. (2006) also identified osteoarthritis as the most common cause of pain (34 per cent) with

Site	Prevalence (%)
Back (unspecified)	24[b]
Lower back	23[a] or 18[b]
Knee	19[a] or 18[b]
Head	15[b]
Leg	14[b]
Shoulder	16[a] or 9[b]
Joints (unspecified)	10[b]
Hip	14[a] or 8[b]
Neck	8[b]
Hand	6[b]
Upper back	6[a] or 5[b]

Table 8.1 Common chronic pains by site in descending order of prevalence
Source: [a]Parsons et al., 2005; [b]Breivik et al., 2006

limbs, joints and the lower back being the most commonly affected. This reflects the age and social status of those participants who took part in the study, the average age being 50 years and over with 61 per cent reporting a significant disability that affected their capacity to work or do other activities. Consequently, the majority was either unemployed or if over retirement age relied heavily on others for support.

The economic effects of chronic pain

In Breivik et al.'s (2006) European study over half of their respondents who had chronic pain were not economically productive. This finding was consistent with earlier work and suggests a relationship between chronic pain and lack of employment and reduced income.

Chronic pain and chronic pain syndrome (CPS)

We have established that there is a significant amount of chronic pain out there but this does not mean that everybody is experiencing pain in the same way. In Breivik et al. (2006) 60 per cent of the respondents felt their pain was adequately managed – despite only 2 per cent seeking help from pain management specialists in the previous year and a third not seeking any help at all. The latter when questioned felt able to manage their pain on their own or had decided to live with their pain. This left 40 per cent complaining of inadequate management of their pain and of these over a fifth had been in pain without an effective treatment for five years or more; overall two-fifths of those with chronic pain felt that they could not function because of their pain.

> **Key point**
>
> Many people with chronic pain are dealing with their problem without help or support from others.

Adapting to chronic pain

Successful adaptation to chronic pain is strongly associated with:

- beliefs of control (Jensen et al., 2007);
- positive problem-solving;

- optimism;
- a commitment to finding solutions;
- a high tolerance for frustration;
- a refusal to consider themselves disabled (Shaw et al., 2001).

Maladapting to chronic pain

Unsuccessful adaption to chronic pain is associated with:

- resting and catastrophizing (Buenaver et al., 2007; Jensen et al., 2007; Turner et al., 2000);
- physical disability and depression (Turner et al., 2000);
- difficulty making decisions (Apkarian et al., 2004; Weiner et al., 2006);
- lack of knowledge or holding harmful beliefs (Jensen et al., 2007);
- poor problem-solving with efforts focused on pain relief and frequently using ill-informed or unproven remedies (Shaw et al., 2001).

Failure to adapt results in passivity, reliance on others, functional loss, raised perception of pain severity, frustration, loss of control and hopelessness. The individual who has not adapted may be basing their values, beliefs, knowledge and attitudes on a misunderstanding of effective pain management (Turk and Monarch, 2002). For example, beliefs that pain is a sign that ongoing damage is occurring, even though it is in fact a steady state that can be improved, will lead to adoption of problem-solving behaviours that work well with acute pain (rest, taking analgesia, seeking help from others) but will lead to disability and adverse coping in chronic pain.

Failure to function, adapt or cope with pain is linked to chronic pain syndrome (Epping-Jordan et al., 1998). Its development appears to reflect a failure to adapt and cope with unimproved symptoms. Individuals perceive the pain as growing worse although this is not always the case. The perception may be linked to the failure in management and the persistent nature of the pain. It is this group, those who have a CPS, which the rest of this chapter focuses on. We do this with the intention of examining attitudes and approaches to helping those people who have not found a method that relieves their chronic pain with the aim of considering ways in which they can be helped.

The development of the syndrome appears to be related to certain factors that interfere with adaption such as depression, fear avoidance (movement), inactivity and relationship problems. Singh and Patel (2005) refer to Sternbach's 6 D's of CPS:

1. *Dramatization* of complaints – where sufferers express pain in ways which appear disproportional, such as moaning and grimacing.
2. *Drug misuse* – often prolonged, which often commences to try to relieve the pain and includes prescription and non-prescription drugs and alcohol.
3. *Dysfunction/disuse* – avoidance of movement or disuse of the affected part resulting in dysfunction.
4. *Dependency* – increasing dependency and withdrawal from social and recreational roles.
5. *Depression* – and other changes in mood.
6. *Disability* – particularly a perception of occupational disability

As a result an individual may present exhibiting a wide range of symptoms (Table 8.2).

Chronic pain syndrome symptoms	
Reduced activity	Anxiety
Impaired sleep	Pain behaviours
Depression	Helplessness
Suicidal ideation	Hopelessness
Social withdrawal	Alcohol abuse
Irritability and fatigue	Medication abuse
Strong somatic focus	Guilt
Memory and cognitive impairment	Relationship problems
Less interest in sex	Poor self-esteem
Misbehaviour by children in the home	Loss of employment
	Fear of movement

Table 8.2 Chronic pain syndrome symptoms

These wide-ranging symptoms demonstrate the global impact chronic pain has on the physical, psychological and social elements of the individual's life. As the pain persists into chronicity, it usually leads to a variety of protective behaviours which further impair function. This fear-avoidance strategy may seem to be a logical process to avoid exacerbating the pain experience (Grotle et al., 2004). Nevertheless, avoiding movement in many causes of chronic pain can lead to worsening of the pain and an increase in the intensity of the fear of moving. If pain is not controlled this fear avoidance impacts markedly on activities of daily living with a reduction in ability or an inability to walk, exercise and lift and therefore fulfil roles such as performing housework or work outside the home (Pincus et al., 2006).

> **Key point**
>
> Ability to function normally is the first casualty of CPS.

For some losing the ability to function normally could result in a loss of paid employment or the need to change occupation or work role. It also has an impact on family relationships and friendships as a consequence of reduced social and sexual activity (Björck-van Dijken et al., 2008). Over half of respondents in Breivik et al.'s (2006) study were less able to sleep and a further 9 per cent said they were no longer able to sleep. Imagine how persistent lack of sleep negatively affects daily life.

Depression

Depression is higher in CPS and its presence at an early stage in the development of chronic pain also predicts the development of CPS (Keeley et al., 2008). In a small study involving 36 patients referred to specialist pain services, 72 per cent of the sample had depression with 86 per cent reporting at least mild depression (Poole et al., 2009). The presence of anxiety in chronic pain sufferers is less well studied than depression but seems to be higher than in the general population. The relationship is unclear as the propensity to be anxious may well have predated the onset of pain. Nevertheless, anxiety can, in some cases, exacerbate pain through increasing muscle tension. These psychological factors, especially depression, significantly influence an individual's perceived quality of life and disability (Borsbo et al., 2009).

Activity 8.1

Read the following case study:

Mr J is a 42-year-old married gentleman with two young children. He has had mechanical low back pain, secondary to an industrial lifting injury, for the past two years. During this time he has been seen by an orthopaedic surgeon, a neurologist, a neurosurgeon, a psychiatrist and a physiotherapist.

All investigations including plain X-rays, MRI and all biochemical tests have been within normal ranges. Despite numerous attendances at his local hospital and general practitioner, he is still in a lot of pain and has become significantly incapacitated. His employers have terminated his employment and he is in the midst of a legal battle in relation to compensation for the injury he sustained at work.

What are the likely effects that this patient's pain may have on him as an individual, and also on his relationships with members of his family?

Impact on spouses, partners and friends

Because of the limiting nature of chronic pain, the loss of an individual's functioning and role impacts on spouses, partners and friends. Therefore, it is important not to forget to assess the impact of someone's chronic pain on significant individuals in the sufferer's life. Schneider (2009: 20) recalls the stories of some who have had to care for those with chronic pain:

> . . . In the doctor's office, I feel like I'm invisible. No one asks me how I'm coping, or what my life is like! . . .

Ever since I was a little girl I dreamed of getting married, having children, and being a housewife. I didn't go to college, since I planned on staying home and raising kids. I married this gorgeous guy with a good career, but after Cal's second back operation, and shortly after my second child was born, it became clear that I needed to get a job. It was overwhelming, taking care of the two babies and him, and working, too. I was very depressed for a long time, and I'd cry and cry when I was alone, so that the kids and Cal wouldn't see. Cal was also very depressed about losing his former life – he was in so much more pain after the surgery. He lost his mobility and his function was minimal. He couldn't be the dad he wanted to be (p. 22).

My depression was grieving for what we lost. I still love him with all my heart, but we haven't had sex for three years [she begins to cry]. We were very sexually active, and it is hard to live with this change. He thinks that if you can't have intercourse, you shouldn't even kiss. I've tried talking with him, but he doesn't seem to understand. I've been thinking maybe if we could go to the counsellor together, but it's difficult to talk about sex with someone else. This loss isn't something that you just get over. I thought I was okay, but it's obvious to me now that I still have strong feelings about these things (p. 24).

Schneider (2009) illustrates through these stories the impact a person's chronic pain has on the partners, life, emotions and relationship with the person with chronic pain.

Maladaptation

The need to treat maladaptation has led to the development of a range of interventions designed to ameliorate or prevent these forms of suffering. Group therapies have been used widely for the management of pain (Keefe et al., 2002), mostly in the form of educational programmes that use instructional methods to tell people what is wrong with them, how treatments work and what they should do about their problems. These have limited clinical benefits and often have retention and maintenance problems. Another form of group working involves cognitive behavioural therapy programmes. These programmes involve experts teaching participants general cognitive and behavioural skills to help them with their chronic pain and do not involve focusing on individual problems in the group setting. While these are beneficial they tend to be very expensive (Keefe et al., 2002). Additionally, social support groups have been set up that may produce some psychological benefits (Keefe et al., 2002). The evidence suggests that multidisciplinary pain management programmes (PMPs) that utilize a cognitive behavioural therapy approach have been effective in reducing the disabling effect of chronic pain by focusing on the restoration of function and improvement in quality of life, rather than a reduction in pain intensity and a reduction in reliance on health services. PMPs incorporate a range of strategies that lie in the realms of personal development, self-awareness, acquisition of knowledge and skills and development of interpersonal skills.

Specific treatment approaches

Reducing the risk of developing chronic pain

Chronic pain syndrome can be very difficult to manage because of its complex history, unclear aetiology and poor response to therapy. As a result prevention would seem to be the best policy, although this is much easier to say than to achieve but it should be possible through a co-ordinated and systematic approach to the problem. The key to this is early referral and intervention by the most appropriate professional in order to ensure that pain is dealt with effectively to prevent chronicity developing.

At the heart of prevention or management is a detailed assessment of the individual's experience of pain. This is something that we cannot emphasize too much. The assessment should not simply focus on the pain but also on its impact. Therefore, a holistic assessment exploring physical, psychological and social functioning of both the individual and immediate family is necessary. In Chapter 4 we emphasized the need to perform a multidimension pain assessment. It is also essential to rule out any underlying cause of the pain that has not been recognized and treated. While this is necessary it is also important not

to subject the individual to unnecessary investigation as this could further increase the psychological impact of the prolonged pain and divert attention from its successful management.

The complex nature of the pain experience requires a multidisciplinary approach. Depending on the chronic pain experience, this may include a wide variety of medical/surgical/nursing specialists and physiotherapists. When asked '*What kind of doctors are you currently seeing specifically about your pain?*' 70 per cent of Breivik et al.'s (2006: 298) sample identified their general or family practitioner. Twenty seven per cent were seeing an orthopaedic surgeon which reflects the origins of the pain experienced by those individuals. Disappointingly, only 2 per cent were currently being managed by a pain management specialist; although when specifically asked if they had ever seen a 'pain management specialist' 23 per cent said they had. The authors suggest that the meaning of this term may vary between countries. In Chapter 6 'Delivering pain management', we considered the state of chronic pain services in the UK and it should be quite clear from the numbers cited in the European pain study (Breivik et al., 2006) that demand currently outstrips supply.

The chronic pain management plan

> **Key point**
>
> Treating chronic pain like acute pain leads to a failure to treat effectively.

As in the previous chapter the key is to have a carefully structured management plan in place. However, in the case of chronic pain, this will be more complex. Good interpersonal skills are important during this process. We previously addressed these issues in Chapter 3 but to summarize there is a need to provide clear communication using patient appropriate terminology, offer logical explanations in an unhurried fashion and clarify perceptions to avoid misunderstandings. As part of this process an aim would be to empower the individual and increase their sense of control.

Any planned programme needs to be evaluated in a systematic way using the most appropriate tools with the outcome of the evaluation documented. This will ensure from assessment to evaluation that each stage of the care of individuals with this multidimensional problem will be effectively communicated within an integrated plan of care. The British Pain Society and Royal College of General Practitioners (2004: 72) recognize the complexities involved in developing such a plan when they set out their five pledges that should be made to people with chronic pain. These are: *'Active involvement in the management of pain; timely assessment of pain; access to appropriate management and support; relevant information and access to adequate resources and facilities'.*

Patients' perceptions

For many individuals their perceptions of the health care system are less than positive with research over time suggesting similar beliefs (Parsons, 1999; Breivik et al., 2006). Individuals recognize the demanding relationship that exists between themselves and their general practitioner. There is often a sense of helplessness as they perceive a lack of interest in the health care professional who does not believe the impact pain is having on their quality of life. This is coupled with doubts as to the professional's ability to manage their pain, or to see their pain as a problem. The following cases illustrate the tensions that can exist.

Activity 8.2

Carefully read the following three statements made by patients with chronic pain and consider what their perceptions are about how their pain is managed:

Patient 1

> To be honest I'm disappointed in my GP. I feel like I only ever got anything when I made a fuss or when I offered to pay myself. See the GP he don't really believe me. The health service now is no good for dealing with my problem great for things like hernias. You know when I was in for this hernia I got to be honest they were marvellous. I was in within a couple of

weeks and I thought I would have to wait months. I thought it was brilliant but with this problem there's nothing there. It's hopeless for dealing with problems like mine you know constant pain.

JB male aged 51 with painful right arm and shoulder for five years (*source*: Parsons, 1999)

Patient 2

> So it started when I had to have surgery on my back, I had to have two titanium bars either side of my spine to keep me up. They were meant to go in through the front and my back but when I went in, they actually needed to go in the back only. But I had ten blood transfusions and was on a tube to breathe in my neck and a chest drain because your lungs automatically go down so they put a chest drain but it's meant to inflate after but mine didn't. My right lung didn't inflate. So they were a bit concerned with that and I was in Intensive Care. But I was very lucky because they only had to go in through the back not the front. So, I've only scars on my back. Any way I had to wear a corset for months and I was housebound for at least 6 months. I couldn't get out of bed and if I did, I had to have two people with me. I couldn't go on my own. I wasn't independent at all. Couldn't get on a bus and I couldn't get into a car or anything. Well a year after this operation I was still having pain as bad as or worse than after the operation. So I went up to London and I said I'm still having this pain and I said look you've got to do something about it. So, he said the operation was a success. I mean how can it be called a success if I'm in such pain and I was better off before? I mean before, I had a hump and it was awkward but I didn't have any pain. Or all the pain I had was tightness here but it wasn't like now. So, I think what was the point in having it? I'm much worse now than when

I have the operation. I mean I'm straighter but what's the point of looking straight if you can't do as much. When the pain is really bad, I think what the hell was the point of me having the operation? So, he said he'd see about me going to a pain clinic.

When I went there to London, I felt that that the doctor up there was proud of the operation. He'd done the surgery and he got the result he wanted but I was left in pain. Technically, he was very pleased. 'Fantastic couldn't be better' and then I was ruining it for him by saying I was in pain so he wasn't interested. [His attitude was] 'Just get on with it'. A number of times when I went up there it were like two train journeys to get there and two to get back. And it cost a lot of money to go to London. And you tell him you're still in pain and oh it's the nerve off hand like and what can you expect and it'll improve but it hasn't. We probably touched a nerve and it's just sparking of pain and there's nothing wrong with that because we've taken blood tests so there's nothing wrong. I went no I don't think so I'm in pain and he wasn't that interested then.

Even my own GP hasn't a clue about what pain I went through and what pain I'm in know. You know even after he's sending me to a pain specialist centre now he does not have a clue. You know when I say I'm in pain he says, 'Well there's your tablets'. Always tablets! The more you take well the more you get worse because I know if I take two now I'd be sleeping for hours. I'd be really tired. Absolutely tired! So I don't think tablets are a good idea.

AH female aged 18 with congenital spinal deformity (*source:* Parsons, 1999)

Patient 3

(in) this system they don't treat the individual. You're a number. You're

numbered: Number one; number two; number 3 and so on. And you go in and they say, 'Oh here's number three! Right have some paracodamol' or something. And that's it! Now each individual's treated the same instead of each individual being examined and then you come to a conclusion. Isn't it? You know I don't know nothing about medicine but I would say that each individual should be examined and then a reasonable conclusion come to for that individual by the medical officer, nurse or doctor or physiotherapist whoever it may be that treat that patient because otherwise you're not accurate. I've definitely had that experience. I've definitely had that experience otherwise them girls in physiotherapy wouldn't have put me on that traction. They wouldn't have put me on that traction if they'd known I'd had a broken bone in the pelvis. See they don't treat you as a person you're just a slab of meat and they wire you up to a machine and they leave you there and you're having electric treatment or traction but they haven't a clue what you really need as they haven't had you're notes.

FS male aged 60 with back and neck pain for 10 years (source: Parsons, 1999)

The experiences and feelings reported by patients in the case studies above can be outlined as follows. First, they all felt that their concerns were not taken seriously by the health professionals who cared for them. Second, they were frustrated that health services designed to treat acute health problems do not help them with their chronic health problem. This is a particular problem for people in chronic pain where the assumption is often made that what works for an acute pain like toothache should work for their chronic pain as well and that the experiences of being in acute pain are the same as those of being in chronic pain. Wall (1999: 176) summarizes as follows *'The reason for this may be that everyone is so familiar with the problem in themselves or in their friends and relatives that the unpleasant effects are ignored'.*

Key point

Attitudes of carers have a profound effect on an individual's treatment outcomes.

These three people quoted also demonstrated a feeling that their interactions with health professionals are

focused on 'getting them sorted out' and treating them as an object rather than treating them as an individual. This feeling was exacerbated by not being kept informed of their condition or the prevalence of a 'doctor or nurse knows best attitude'. Consequently, it is important that both patients and professionals are clear about the nature of the problem and the goals that care hopes to achieve. This will overcome many of the frustrations highlighted above. The importance of this is illustrated in the following activity.

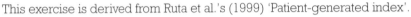

Activity 8.3

This exercise is derived from Ruta et al.'s (1999) 'Patient-generated index'.

Ask five patient/clients or families what problems their pain is causing or has caused them and how they want to tackle them using the following chart.

Stage 1 involves identifying up to six problems that your patient/client or family has and wishes to have help with.

Stage 2 requires the patient/client or their family to score each area or activity they have problems with out of 100 using the scoring system below. They should have up to six scores out of 100–1 for each problem.

100 Exactly as you would like to be
90 Close to how you would like to be
80 Very good but not how you would like to be
70 Good but not how you would like to be
60 Between fair and good
50 Fair
40 Between poor and fair
30 Poor but not the worst you could imagine
20 Very poor but not the worst you could imagine
10 Close to the worst you could imagine
0 The worst you could imagine

Stage 3 introduces the idea of spending points on their problem. A point refers to how much they want this problem dealt with. They have 60 points and must allocate them so that the total number of points spent does not exceed this number. They can choose to spend some points on all other aspects of their life if they wish.

Example of how to use Ruta et al.'s (1999) patient-generated index:

Stage 1	Stage 2	Stage 3
Area/activity	**Score each area/activity out 100**	**Spend your 60 points between the different areas**
Sleeping	75	15
Going to the toilet	30	8
Playing with children	60	10
Sex	40	7
Pain	50	5
Housework	25	5
All other aspects of your life not mentioned above	**You must fill in this box**	10

Now use the following template to make an assessment on each of your five patients:

Stage 1	Stage 2	Stage 3
Area/activity	**Score each area/activity out 100**	**Spend your 60 points between the different areas**
All other aspects of your life not mentioned above	**You must fill in this box**	

The purpose of this activity is to focus on what patients have decided is their priority for pain management. If you are patient-centred in your approach you should be able to match each area with your own priorities. If we had asked you to list your main priority you may have put down 'Freedom from pain'; if this then matched your patients' criteria then you will have done well; however, often people have different requirements.

In the example we have used a woman with a young family who has chronic pelvic pain. Although pain is ranked high as an initial score of 50 there are two other areas that cause the patient more concern; these are playing with her children and sleep. However, when we ask her to identify those problems she needs the most help with using the spending of points, we can see that there are other areas she would rather we concentrated our time on. For this lady getting adequate sleep is seen as a high priority and she wants to spend a quarter of her 60 points on this. Next is playing with her children and she awards a hefty 10 points to this specific activity. Going to the toilet and sex follow with pain and housework given a lower priority. This is an important exercise because if you are going to meet the biopsychosocial needs of your patients you must focus on those problems they wish you to tackle.

Did all five of your patients prioritize the same problems or activities? This can be another problem. Just because you might be patient-centred with one patient that does not mean that you are with the next. Failure to recognize this can lead to conflict.

Dealing with pain behaviours

Combating fear avoidance strategies

The fear-avoidance model of chronic pain (Fig. 8.2) offers an explanation for how chronic pain can develop in some individuals. It suggests that following injury the pain experience can be interpreted in one of two ways. For those who do not perceive the pain as being threatening, they rapidly confront the pain with modifying activities that lead to recovery. Individuals who perceive the pain as a threat, have a predisposition to this perception and excessively worry, that is, catastrophizing, suffer pain-related fear which leads to avoidance strategies and hypervigilance. Over time, individuals can develop a distorted view that nothing is going to help their pain and may give up on treatments believing nothing can work. This can lead to disuse, depression and disability. This further exacerbates the pain experience and so a vicious cycle is perpetuated.

Assessment needs to consider all the stages in the cycle outlined in Fig. 8.2 before an individualized care plan can be made. Fear avoidance, particularly of movement, is the most destructive health behaviour seen in chronic pain. It can lead to withdrawal from social, physical and psychological activity. Those who

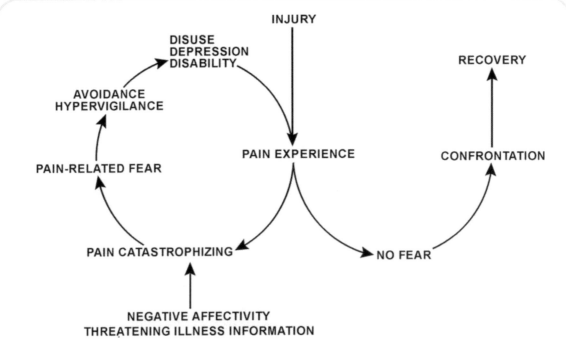

Figure 8.2 The fear-avoidance model of chronic pain.
Source: from Vlaeyen, J.W. and Linton, S.J. (2000) 'Fear avoidance and its consequences in musculoskeletal pain: a state of the art', *Pain*, 85(3): 329. This figure has been reproduced with permission of the International Association for the Study of Pain® (IASP®). The figure may not be reproduced for any other purpose without permission.

avoid activity have the biggest incidence of disability and distress (McCracken and Samuel, 2007) and they require a great deal of sensitivity in developing a plan of care. It usually leads to a variety of protective behaviours which further impair functioning; one that is commonly experienced is activity cycling.

McCracken and Samuel (2007) performed a study on 276 individuals with chronic pain which compared three activities: avoidance, pacing and confronting. Avoidance was defined as inactivity because of pain or not engaging in activity that causes pain to increase. Pacing was defined as using repeated rest breaks or working more slowly in order to complete tasks and confronting as pushing to get things done despite the pain or spending too much time on a task and experiencing increased pain later. They were able to identify four distinct strategies:

1. *Avoiders:* exhibit moderately high avoidance, with high levels of pacing when they are not in pain and low confrontation when they are in pain.
2. *Extreme cyclers:* demonstrate high confronting, with frequent pacing which leads to increased pain and prolonged avoidance.
3. *Medium cyclers:* display high levels of confronting and moderate pacing and avoidance.
4. *Doers:* portray high levels of activity despite pain with low levels of trying to manage pain by pacing or avoiding – they are more accepting of their pain.

In this study avoiders demonstrated the lowest physical activity and highest physical disability and anxiety, but they were closely followed by extreme cyclers who demonstrated an increased tendency to avoid when they were in pain (McCracken and Samuel, 2007).

Early support may need to focus on underlying fears about the nature of the pain experience and reassurance that the activities proposed will not exacerbate the problem. This can be a difficult stage in management but one that can be overcome. If this is not achieved early in the plan then it is unlikely that avoidance strategies can be diminished.

Activity cycling

The variation in pain score over time can be more easily seen in Fig. 8.3 and Table 8.3.

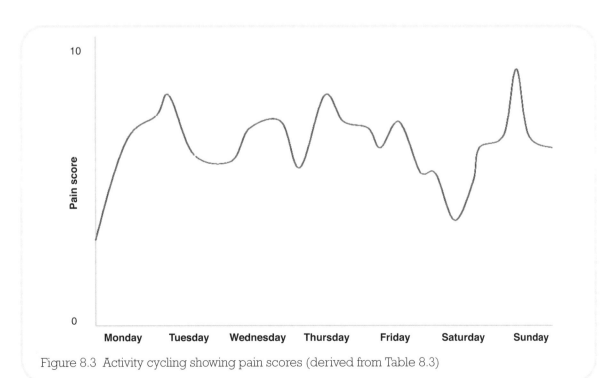

Figure 8.3 Activity cycling showing pain scores (derived from Table 8.3)

Monday	Tuesday	Wednesday	Thursday
Woke up with moderate pain 4/10	Pain very severe this morning about 9/10	Pain still severe 9/10 again	Pain still severe but seems easier 7/10
Food shopping in morning	Couldn't get out of bed	Didn't sleep last night, painkillers no good.	Managed to get to sleep about 3 am.
Still have moderate pain 4/10	Felt tearful	Called GP this morning as couldn't get out of bed	Tidied house before GP came – back now worse, pain 9/10
Mowed the lawn in the afternoon (front and back)	Got up this afternoon about 1 pm, very stiff, pain 7/10	He won't come until tomorrow	GP gave me an injection
Pain worse 7/10	Made lunch, couldn't stand for more than 2 minutes at a time	Stayed in bed all day	Pain 4/10
Cooked meal for family, difficulty in standing	Children had to cook evening meal	Pain 8/10	Did ironing and cooked a meal
Pain severe in the evening 8/10	Pain score at bedtime still 7/10	Rest of day very tired and irritable	Pain 7/10 in evening

Friday	Saturday	Sunday	
Pain 7/10 again	Woke up this morning with moderate pain 4/10	Pain very severe again 9/10	
Argument with Mike (husband)	Went shopping with children, and then to the cinema	Mike cooked Sunday dinner	
Made me get up, pain 8/10 called pain clinic in tears, spoke to nurse, must do some gentle exercise.	Found it difficult to walk in the afternoon but put on a brave face, pain 7/10	Stayed in bed till 2 pm, pain 7/10	
Couldn't do all stretches but did most, felt better in myself	Had to lie down in the evening, pain 7/10	Thought about doing exercises but too stiff to move	
Tired		Watched TV in the evening	
Pain 6/10		Pain score 7/10	

Table 8.3 Extract from a pain diary showing features of activity cycling

You can see that doing high levels of activity when the patient's visual analogue scale (VAS) score was low (Table. 8.3) had a directly adverse effect on her pain because she overdid things. It is important at this stage to distinguish between an 'extreme cycler' and a 'doer', because while both might well experience the same increase in pain, the emotional and help-seeking responses to this increase would differ. A doer would not experience the same level of distress and help-

seeking behaviour, which is manifested in the diary as getting children to prepare meals or calling the GP or pain clinic.

The approach to fear avoidance is to introduce pacing. However, we can see in this diary that there is some pacing. The problem is that this is not effectively structured and it leads to a worsening pain problem. If not addressed this can lead to people progressively doing less, losing body condition and not being able to plan ahead because of uncertainty about their pain and allowing others to do things for them (McLaren and McLaren, 2010). Pacing strategies focus on allaying underlying fears about the cause of pain and reassurance that the activities proposed will not exacerbate the problem. This can be a difficult stage in management but one that can be overcome. If this is not achieved early in the plan then it is unlikely that avoidance strategies can be diminished. Activities are introduced at a manageable and slow pace so that short-term goals are achieved. The nature of the activity will depend on the site of the pain. As activity increases, strength flexibility and endurance will increase while pain will decrease. A pacing approach to inactivity is as follows:

- avoids excessive activity which leads to excess rest;
- uses the same amount of activity on every day;
- uses activity that is of a low to moderate intensity;
- schedules increasing activity and exercises;
- avoids the temptation to do more on a good day;
- improves condition and physical endurance.

This is achieved through a structured pain management plan that sets goals, is monitored closely and requires compliance in order to extinguish avoidance behaviours. The plan must be functional and relevant to the person in pain in order to improve their conditions (McCracken and Samuel, 2006). One way of achieving this is to work towards medium- and long-term 'valued directions' (McLaren and McLaren, 2010), chosen by the person in pain. Valued directions are shaped by considerations about the sort of person they want to be and involve ideas about personal growth and their relationships with others, rather than continually striving to cure a chronic health problem; Ruta's patient-generated index is one way of eliciting these valued directions.

Dealing with anxiety, depression and anger

These three aversive emotions are often associated with chronic pain and their presence is usually indicative that some degree of CPS is involved. The response to dealing with these problems depends on the severity of the condition and, especially in the case of anxiety and depression, may need to be treated before any specific pain treatment is given. In mild to moderate cases there may be no need to treat anxiety or depression with medication or medication can be used alongside physical or cognitive approaches.

Anxiety can respond to appropriate relaxation techniques as part of an overall pain syndrome intervention programme and depression can be helped using structured increases in activity, as seen in pacing, alongside goals aimed at improving interpersonal skills such as assertiveness. Similarly, anger can be managed through a mixture of goal-setting and good interpersonal communication. Key to this is accepting a person's report of their pain. Much of their anger stems from past carers indicating that the pain was 'all in their head', or that it 'had no physical basis'. One approach to dealing with anger involves anger expression through an exercise involving written emotional disclosure. Graham et al. (2008) demonstrated that expressing anger towards a person who had upset them or towards the pain itself, by writing a letter addressed to that person or their pain which expressed their strong feelings, helped people with chronic pain find meaning. This process lessened their anger and moderated their mood.

Summary

This chapter has considered chronic pain as a complex multidimensional problem that has a heavy and malign impact on a person's life. We have deliberately focused on the lived experience of chronic pain as in our opinion how someone adapts to their pain will determine their ability to function and their quality of life. We acknowledge that many people with chronic pain do adapt and are able to live full lives but these are not the people who are routinely seen in pain clinics. We also acknowledge that there are treatments that can ameliorate and occasionally remove chronic pain and we have deliberately chosen not to examine them as many of these do not last for a lifetime and can generate their own problems. Instead, we have looked at the experience of having CPS. Chronic pain syndrome is undoubtedly a challenge for health carers because of its complex history, unknown aetiology and poor response to treatment. It is an even greater challenge to those who have to spend every day living with it; both sufferers and their loved ones.

After reading this chapter you should:

- have an understanding of the extent and nature of chronic pain;
- recognize that some people struggle to adapt to chronic pain;
- realize that helping people with chronic pain involves a holistic approach and should not just focus on the physical aspects of their pain.

Reflective activity

As a conclusion to this chapter consider how knowledge of this theory will help you in your future practice. Try to be specific and use the following points/questions as a guide.

- *State* which elements of the chapter will help you in your future practice. For example, you might consider how a person adapts to chronic pain influences their experience of pain.
- *Elaborate:* be specific in terms of how this knowledge and understanding can be used in practice. As an example consider how attitudes to people with chronic pain have a big influence on adaptation. Are you aware of your own attitudes to people with chronic pain?
- *Give examples:* of care events which would benefit from what you have learnt. Often the first meeting with someone in chronic pain shapes the ongoing relationship. How would you deal with someone who displays CPS pain behaviours?

What are the *implications* if you change the way you practise. Do you need to change your attitude and approach to people with chronic pain? What skills do you need to deal with the complex problems seen in CPS?

You may prefer to use a reflective model such as Gibbs's (1988) to guide your reflection (see Appendix at the end of this book). It may help to consider specific examples as the starting point; for example, a patient's pain behaviours seem to be incongruent to their actual injuries. When analysing the situation draw on this chapter's theory to support your discussion and demonstrate your understanding. As a result your reflection should examine the key principles:

- Chronic pain syndrome is a real health problem affecting many sufferers.
- A structured approach can resolve chronic pain problems.
- An approach aimed at changing behaviours must use goals that are personally relevant and valued by the person with chronic pain.

References

Apkarian, A.V., Sosa, Y., Krauss, B.R., Thomas, P.S., Fredrickson, B.E., Levy, R.E. et al. (2004) Chronic pain patients are impaired on an emotional decision-making task, *Pain*, 108: 129–36.

Björck-van Dijken, C., Fjellman-Wiklund, A. and Hildingsson, C. (2008) Low back pain, lifestyle factors and physical activity: a population-based study, *Journal of Rehabilitation Medicine*, 40: 864–869.

Borsbo, B., Peolsson, M. and Gerdle, B. (2009) The complex interplay between pain intensity, depression, anxiety and catastrophising with respect to quality of life and disability, *Disability & Rehabilitation*, 31(19): 1605–13.

Breivik, H., Collett, C., Ventafridda, V., Cohen, R. and Gallacher, D. (2006) Survey of chronic pain in Europe: prevalence, impact on daily life, and treatment, *European Journal of Pain*, 10: 287–333.

British Pain Society and Royal College of General Practitioners (2004) *A Practical Guide to the Provision of Chronic Pain Services for Adults in Primary Care*. London: The British Pain Society and the Royal College of General Practitioners.

Buenaver, L.F., Edwards, R.R. and Haythornthwaite, J.A. (2007) Pain-related catastrophizing and perceived social responses: inter-relationships in the context of chronic pain, *Pain*, 127, 234–42.

Epping-Jordan, J.E., Wahlgren, D.R., Williams, R.A., Pruitt, S.D., Slater, M.A., Patterson, T.L., Grant, I., Webster, J.S. and J.H.A. (1998) Transition to chronic pain in men with low back pain: predictive relationships among pain intensity, disability, and depressive symptoms, *Health Psychology*, 17(5): 421–7.

Gibbs, G. (1988) *Learning by Doing: A Guide to Teaching and Learning Methods*. Oxford: Further Education Unit, Oxford Polytechnic.

Graham, J., Lobel, M., Glass, P. and Lokshina, I. (2008) Effects of written anger expression in chronic pain patients: making meaning from pain, *Journal of Behavioral Medicine*, 31(3), 201–12.

Grotle, M., Vøllestad, N.K., Veierød, M.B. and Brox, J.I. (2004) Fear-avoidance beliefs and distress in relation to disability in acute and chronic low back pain, *Pain*, 112(3): 343–52.

Gureje, O., Von Korff, M., Simon, G.E. and Gater, R. (1998) Persistent pain and well being: a World Health Organization study in primary care, *Journal of the American Medical Association*, 280: 147–51.

Hardt, J., Jacobsen, C., Goldberg, J., Nickel, R. and Buchwald, D. (2008) Prevalence of chronic pain in a representative sample in the United States, *Pain Medicine*, 9(7): 803–12.

International Association for the Study of Pain (IASP) (1986) Classification of chronic pain: descriptions of chronic pain syndromes and definitions of pain terms, *Pain*, Supplement: 3) S1–S225.

——— (2006–2007) Global Year Against Pain: 2006–2007 Campaign – Pain in Older Persons. Available at: www.iasp-pain.org/AM/Template.cfm?Section=2006_2007_Pain_in_Older_Persons1&Template=/CM/HTMLDisplay.cfm&ContentID=4637 (accessed January 2010).

International Association for the Study of Pain (IASP) European Federation of IASP Chapters (EFIC) (2004–2005a) *Factsheet 4A: Unrelieved pain is a major global healthcare problem*. Available online at www.iasp-pain.org/AM/Template. cfm?Section=Press_Release&Template=/CM/ContentDisplay.cfm&ContentID=2908 (accessed January 2010).

——— (2004–2005b) *Factsheet 5: Why pain control matters in a world full of killer diseases*. Available online at: www.iasp-pain.org/AM/Template.cfm?Section=Press_Release&Template=/CM/ ContentDisplay.cfm&ContentID=2911 (accessed January 2010).

Jensen, M.P., Turner, J.A. and Romano, J.M. (2007) Changes after multidisciplinary pain treatment in patient pain beliefs and coping are associated with concurrent changes in patient functioning, *Pain*, 131(1–2): 38–47.

Keefe, F.J., Beaupre, P.M., Gil, K.M., Rumble, M.E. and Aspnes, A.K. (2002) Group therapy for patients with chronic pain, in D. C. Turk and R. J. Gatchel (eds) (2002) *Psychological Approaches to Pain Management: A Practitioner's Handbook*, pp. 590 New York: Guilford Press.

Keeley, P., Creed, F., Tomenson, B., Todd, C., Borglin, G. and Dickens, C. (2008) Psychosocial predictors of health-related quality of life and health service utilisation in people with chronic low back pain, *Pain*, 135(1–2): 142–50.

McCracken, L.M. and Samuel, V.M. (2007) The role of avoidance, pacing, and other activity patterns in chronic pain, *Pain*, 130(1–2): 119–25.

McLaren, E. and McLaren, R. (2010) Psychological approaches to managing chronic back pain, in A. Clarke, A. Jones, M. O'Malley and R. McLaren (eds) *ABC of Spinal Disorders*, pp. 52–7. Chichester: BMJ Publishing/Wiley-Blackwell.

Ospini, M. and Harstall, C. (2002) *Prevalence of Chronic Pain: An Overview*. Alberta Heritage Foundation for Medical Research: HTA 29 Health Technology Assessment.

Parsons, G. (1999) A comparison of patient expectations of a chronic pain service with commissioner's expectations of outcomes. Unpublished MSc dissertation, UWCM, Cardiff.

Parsons, S., Underwood, M., Breen, A., Foster, N., Pincus, T. and Vogel, S. (2005) What is the prevalence of chronic muskuloskeletal pain in the community? *Journal of Bone Joint Surgery* (British volume), 87b B (Supplement: II) 207.

Pincus, T., Vogel, S., Burton, A.K., Santos, R. and Field, A.P. (2006) Fear avoidance and prognosis in back pain: a systematic review and synthesis of current evidence [systematic review] *Arthritis & Rheumatism*, 54(12), 3999–4010.

Poole, H., White, S., Blake, C.m Murphy, P. and Bramwell, R. (2009) Depression in chronic pain patients: prevalence and measurement, *Pain Practice*, 9(3): 173–80.

Ruta, D.A., Garratt, A.M. and Russell, I.T. (1999) Patient centred assessment of quality of life for patients with four common conditions, *Quality Health Care*, 8(1): 22–9.

Schneider, J.P. (2009) Living with chronic pain: the effect on the partner, *The Pain Practitioner*, 19: 1, 20, 22, 24, 26, 30.

Shaw, W.S., Feuerstein, M., Haufler, A.J., Berkowitz, S.M. and Lopez, M.S. (2001) Working with low back pain: problem-solving orientation and function, *Pain*, 93: 129–37.

Singh, M.K. and Patel, J. (2005) Chronic pain syndrome, *eMedicine*, October. Available online at www.emedicine.medscape.com/article/310834-overview (accessed December 2009).

Turk, D.C. and E.S. Monarch (2002) *Biopsychosocial perspectives on chronic pain*, in D.C. Turk and R.J. Gatchel (eds) *Psychological Approaches to Pain Management: A practitioner's Handbook* (p. 590), New York: Guildford Press.

Turner, J.A., Jensen, M.P. and Romano, J.M. (2000) Do beliefs, coping, and catastrophizing independently predict functioning in patients with chronic pain? *Pain*, 1–2: 115–25.

Vlaeyen, J.W. and Linton, S.J. (2000) Fear-avoidance and its consequences in chronic musculoskeletal pain: a state of the art, *Pain*, 85(3): 317–32.

Wall, P. (1999) *Pain: The Science of Suffering*. London: Wiedenfeld & Nicholson.

Weiner, D.K., Rudy, T.E., Morrow, L., Slaboda, J. and Lieber, S. (2006) The relationship between pain, neuropsychological performance, and physical function in community-dwelling older adults with chronic low back pain, *Pain Medicine*, 7(1): 60–70.

9

Pain management in palliative care

Maria Parry

Chapter contents

Introduction
Definition of key concepts
   Supportive care
   Terminal care
Life-limiting conditions
Defining pain in life-limiting conditions
Cancer pain
Multiple sclerosis (MS) and pain
HIV/AIDS and pain
Pain assessment
Pain assessment tools in palliative care
   Factors to consider during assessment
Psychosocial factors influencing the pain
experience
   Consequences of pain
Barriers to pain assessment and management
Pharmacological and non-pharmacological
management of pain in palliative care

Approaches to pain management in
patients who have cancer
Drug management
The analgesic ladder
   Modification of pathological processes
   Interruption to pain pathways
   Non-pharmocological treatment:
      psychological and physical approaches
   Complementary therapies
Immobilization
Rehabilitation – modification of daily
activities
Summary
Reflective activity
References
Further reading

Introduction

In comparison to many other specialities in health care, palliative care has a relatively short history. The term 'palliative care' has been understood to be different things during this time. This transition in terms of definition has reflected its growing maturity as a speciality in health care and acceptance within the multidisciplinary team. However, this growth has also brought with it confusion among practitioners. As Payne et al. (2002) suggests the terminology used and the definitions of these terms are poorly understood. As a result, this chapter explores our understanding of key concepts before examining pain management in palliative care.

A chapter such as this is bound to have its limitations. First, we focus on one aspect of care management and in effect separate it from the complexity that is the care of individuals with a life-limiting condition. As a result, we emphasize that the management of pain should be considered within the holistic assessment and care of the individual as the experience of pain will undoubtedly impact on other problems the individual is experiencing and likewise those problems on the pain experience. Second, we restrict ourselves to a limited number of conditions when illustrating the principles of pain management in palliative care. We ask you to consider these principles in relationship to other life-limiting conditions that you may come across in your professional and personal lives.

There are five broad areas that are covered in this chapter. They are:

1. key concepts in palliative care;
2. exploring the concept of pain in relation to specific life-limiting conditions;
3. the causes of pain in the selected life-limiting conditions;
4. pain assessment in palliative care;
5. management of pain in palliative care.

As a result the following objectives will be achieved:

- Define the key concepts of palliative care.
- Identify the possible causes of pain in three life-limiting conditions.
- Consider the role of assessment and the appropriateness of using pain assessment tools in the management of life-limiting conditions.
- Suggest a range of pharmacological and non-pharmacological approaches to pain management.

Definition of key concepts

Palliative care is synonymous with holistic multi-disciplinary care yet there are some terms which remain problematic in everyday use. Three terms that are often used interchangeably are 'palliative care', 'supportive care' and 'terminal care'.

Activity 9.1

What do you understand by these three terms? Think about their similarities and differences. List the key components of each in the table below. Once you have done that, note the similarities and differences to the other two terms.

Term	Key components	Similarities or differences to the other two terms
Palliative care		
Supportive care		

Term	Key components	Similarities or differences to the other two terms
Terminal care		

The World Health Organization (WHO, 1990: 11) defined palliative care as '*Active total care of patients and their families by a multi professional team when the patient's disease is no longer responsive to curative treatment*'.

Five years later the National Council for Hospice and Specialist Palliative Care Services (NCHSPCS, 1995: 2), now called the National Council for Palliative Care (NCPC), offered another definition:

> *Palliative care is the holistic care of patients with advanced progressive illness. Management of pain and other symptoms and provision of psychological, social, and spiritual support is paramount. The goal of palliative care is achievement of the best quality of life for patients and their families. Many aspects of palliative care are also applicable earlier in the course of the illness in conjunction with other treatments*

The above definition stresses three key components of palliative care:

- active total care (holistic care, in the newer definition);
- not responsive to curative treatment;
- quality of life.

In considering the phrase 'active total care', it is useful to split the term into two parts, namely active and total. *Active care* would be care that is proactive and not reactive. It is care that anticipates problems, and provides relief from distressing symptoms. Active care demonstrates attributes that are considered life-affirming. *Total care* would integrate the physical, spiritual, social and emotional aspects of care, holistic care as we would describe this today.

The phrase, *not responsive to curative treatment* indicates that the condition cannot be cured. However, it does not mean that it cannot be treated. Treatment may not be able to significantly increase life expectancy, but could do much to alleviate distressing symptoms by improving quality of life, enabling an individual to live as full and active life as possible.

Quality of life refers to care that respects the individual as a person first and a patient second. Ensuring consistency and continuity in the provision and delivery of care is one of its key principles. Another key principle would be that of facilitating the individual to live as active a life as possible, despite the constraints caused by their illness.

Supportive care

The second term was that of 'supportive care'. Everyone facing life-threatening illness will need some degree of supportive care in addition to treatment for their condition. Supportive care is an 'umbrella' term for all services, both generalist and specialist, that may be required to support people with life-limiting disease and also their carers. It should not be seen as a response to a stage of disease, but is based on a theory that people will have a need for supportive care from the time that the diagnosis is first raised. The National Institute for Health and Clinical Excellence (NICE, 2004) has defined supportive care for people with cancer. The principles highlighted in this definition could be applied to all life-limiting conditions.

Supportive care can be defined as that which:

> ... *helps the patient and their family to cope with cancer and treatment of it – from pre-diagnosis, through the process of diagnosis and treatment, to cure, continuing illness or death and into bereavement. It helps the patient to maximise the benefits of treatment and to live as well as possible with the effects of the disease. It is given equal priority alongside diagnosis and treatment.*
>
> (NICE, 2004: 18)

Supportive care should be fully integrated with diagnosis and treatment and encompasses:

- Self/help and support
- User involvement
- Information giving
- Psychological support
- Symptom control
- Social support
- Rehabilitation
- Complementary therapies
- Spiritual support
- End of life and bereavement care

(NICE, 2004: 18)

Supportive care is not a distinct specialty, but an umbrella term and it is the responsibility of all health and social care professionals delivering care. It requires a spectrum of skills, extending from foundation skills to highly specific expertise and experience. In principle, supportive care could be viewed as the same as palliative care. The palliative care approach recommends that all patients facing a progressive, life-limiting disease would benefit from a palliative care approach to their care. It should be an integral part of *all* practice, and should not be exclusive to dedicated palliative care centres

Terminal care

The third term suggested was 'terminal care'. This is a large component of palliative care which remains focused on the last days of life. It may be classed as the terminal phase or care of the dying. It continues to be thought of as synonymous with palliation, often being confused as one and the same, while it is essentially a separate component of the overall palliative

care journey, but one which demands expertise in its own right.

> **Key point**
>
> Terminal care is associated with the last days of life. It forms a part of the palliative care journey, but in itself is not palliative care.

The WHO (2004) suggest that although for many patients with a life-limiting progressive illness, survival chances have greatly improved, for some within society they can remain poor, and this relative risk is often related to geographical, cultural and environmental factors, age and stage of disease. The WHO (2004) go on to suggest that while the differences between diseases and survival chances differ, the problems at the end of life however are all too similar. Therefore to predict when a patient is or has entered this phase can prove useful. This has historically been difficult to predict and one which can be misjudged. Three typical illness trajectories have been described for patients with progressive chronic illness: cancer, organ failure, and the frail elderly or dementia trajectory (Murray et al., 2005). This has been supported with the development of the Gold Standards Framework (GSF) (2006) prognostic indicator guide, which does go some way in assisting in this problematic area.

Life-limiting conditions

As the name suggests, life-limiting conditions are ones that reduce life expectancy in an individual when compared to others of a similar age and gender, and who live in comparative social and financial circumstances but who are not diagnosed with the condition.

Life-limiting conditions can affect individuals at all ages; the incidence is high in some and extremely rare in others and can affect all body systems. Table 9.1 lists just some of these conditions.

Pain can be experienced in all these conditions. For some the pain experience will be an overwhelming problem; in others the pain may be relatively mild. It is not our intention to try and address the pain management of all life-limiting conditions; we focus on

Examples of life-limiting conditions	
Cancer	Irreversible organ failure
Multiple sclerosis	Cystic fibrosis
HIV	Batten's disease
Motor neurone disease	Muscular dystrophy
Chronic obstructive pulmonary disease	Severe cerebral palsy
Cerebrovascular accident	Multiple disabilities following brain or spinal cord injury
End stage renal disease	
Dementia	
End stage liver disease	
Congestive heart failure	

Table 9.1 Examples of potentially life-limiting conditions

some specific examples that illustrate the complexity that is involved in managing this problem.

Defining pain in life-limiting conditions

In Chapter 1 we examined a number of ways that pain can be defined and classified and so this discussion will not be repeated here. Nevertheless, in life-limiting conditions the management of pain can be a complex process in that there may be multiple origins of the pain, both somatic and visceral; it may be a mix of acute and chronic; nociceptive and neuropathic, and related to the pathophysiological processes associated with the underlying condition and the psychosocial impact of the diagnosis. To add further complexity to the situation, the pain experienced by the individual may be as a result of the therapy they are receiving and is therefore iatrogenic.

As a result it is inappropriate to consider pain in life-limiting conditions as a singular entity; likewise to term the pain experience *palliative pain*. As discussed elsewhere in this book each individual requires a holistic assessment and reassessment so that a nature of the pain experience can be adequately identified and described. It is only then can we define the nature of the pain and put in place appropriate supportive care.

To further explore the nature of the pain experi-

ence in life-limiting conditions, the focus here is on three specific diagnoses – cancer, multiple sclerosis (MS) and HIV.

Cancer pain

Cancer Research UK (2009) report that in 2007 there were 155 484 deaths from cancer in the UK illustrating the potential size of the problem that would need managing. Earlier work by Kaye (1999) suggests that 30 per cent of cancer patients suffer pain. This emphasizes the importance of accurate assessment, rather than assumption. Faull and Woof (2002) place the figure as high as 50 per cent. Twycross and Wilcock (2001) give figures that one-third of cancer patients have a single pain, one-third two pains and similarly one-third having three or more pains. The WHO (1996) agrees with this assessment.

The last 20 years have seen many advances in medicine, cancer care being no exception. This has in part been due to the growing amount of research in this area and the use of clinical trials for new drugs that may be used as analgesics. Pain is an important symptom as it can be a dominant symbol of the disease which often makes a person seek medical advice.

Establishing the cause of the pain in the patient with cancer is a crucial element in the whole process as this will help in its management (SIGN, 2008). Pain in the cancer patient (see Fig. 9.1) can be caused by:

- the cancer itself;
- related to cancer treatment;
- related to a concurrent disorder;
- complications related to the cancer.

The WHO (1996: 5) also make the important distinction that a patient with advancing disease can have more than one pain which can be from several of the categories listed above. They also specify a series of pain syndromes that are unique to cancer, suggesting that in order to gain a correct diagnosis an awareness of these syndromes is essential.

Multiple sclerosis (MS) and pain

There are an estimated 100 000 people with a diagnosis of MS in the UK (Multiple Sclerosis Society, 2009) and the course of the disease is unpredictable (Plumb, 2006) with, for some people, a period of remission and relapse and for others a more progressive pattern. The Multiple Sclerosis Society (2009) have suggested that it was not until the mid-1980s that many people considered MS to be a condition that could result in pain as a symptom. Now it is generally accepted that MS can cause pain with estimates of 80 per cent of patients with MS having pain (Archibald et al., 1994). Although the nature of the pain experience is not predictable, it can vary between an acute episode lasting for a very short period, or more prolonged. The pain can be intense or an ache that persists and is disruptive.

MS is a chronic disease of the central nervous system (the brain and spinal cord), usually being diagnosed in individuals between 20 and 40 years of

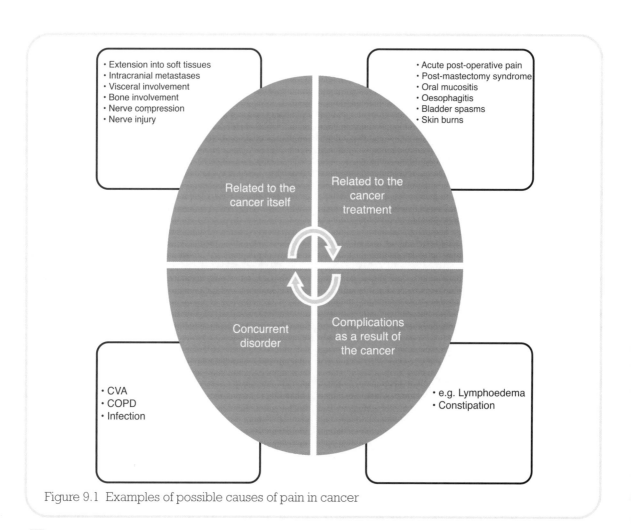

Figure 9.1 Examples of possible causes of pain in cancer

age. For reasons that are not fully understood, damage occurs to the myelin sheath that protects the nerves and aids transmission of messages. When myelin is damaged, the transmission of messages from the brain and spinal cord to the rest of the body is disrupted, interfering with the body's normal ability to function. One of the results of this disruption may be pain along with a wide range of other symptoms such as loss of balance, bladder and bowel dysfunction, fatigue, disruption of memory and cognitive skills, alteration in mood, muscle spasm, tremor, speech and swallowing difficulties, which all impact on social functioning. As a result the pain experience has to be considered within a complex presentation of problems which can make assessment challenging.

MS can cause pain either directly, due to nerve damage, or indirectly, due to MS symptoms, their treatment, or other causes (Figure 9.2). Not everybody with MS experiences pain and it is unlikely that anyone will experience all the types of pain.

Neuropathic pain in MS can also present in a number of ways. Listed below are examples of types and their possible presentations:

- *Trigeminal neuralgia:* an intense, sharp, stabbing facial pain. The pain is usually short-lived, but can leave behind a longer-lasting aching or burning. It is a relatively rare sensation in MS.
- *L'Hermitte's sign:* a sudden, electric-shock-like sensation that spreads into the arms or legs, often triggered when the neck is bent forward, or after a cough or sneeze.
- *Optic neuritis:* visual problems are sometimes, but not always, accompanied by pain when the eye is moved.
- *Tonic spasms:* this sort of painful spasm causes legs or arms to bend or shoot out unexpectedly. They usually last for seconds rather than minutes.
- *Dysesthetic extremity pain:* tingling, numbness, shivering, burning, pins-and-needles or 'creeping pain'. These sensations might come out of the blue or be triggered by super-sensitive skin; for

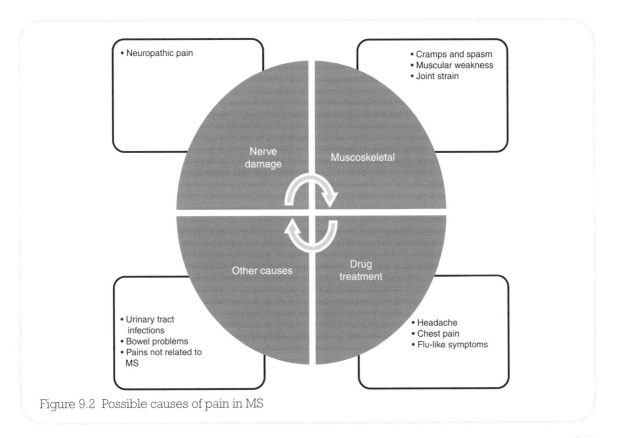

Figure 9.2 Possible causes of pain in MS

Stage	Characteristics
1. Asymptomatic	Asymptomatic, or short flu-like illness Persistent generalized lymphadenopathy
2. Mild symptoms	Moderate unexplained weight loss, recurrent respiratory tract infections, herpes zoster; oral ulceration; dermatitis; fungal nail infections
3. Advanced symptoms	Examples: Unexplained severe weight loss; unexplained chronic diarrhoea; pulmonary tuberculosis and other severe respiratory infections; unexplained anaemia, neutropenia and/or thrombocytopenia
4. Severe symptoms	Examples: HIV wasting syndrome; recurrent pneumonia and other respiratory infections; chronic herpes simplex; kaposi sarcoma; HIV encephalopathy; lymphoma

Table 9.2 Clinical staging of HIV disease

example, where just the lightest of touches feels unpleasant or painful.

- *Girdling, banding or squeezing:* 'a tight band', or constricting pain, usually around the trunk of the body.

HIV/AIDS and pain

In light of the new developments in treatments for HIV, the life span of patients with a HIV diagnosis is increasing; this also means that maintaining and controlling symptoms such as pain is vital for a potentially longer time span. In 2008, there were at least 7370 new diagnoses of HIV contributing to a cumulative total of 102 333 reported by the end of 2008. Eighteen thousand five hundred and sixty people diagnosed with HIV have died and of those at least 80 per cent following an AIDS diagnosis (AVERT, 2009). Pain has a profound negative impact both on physical and psychological functioning and overall quality of life. People with HIV can experience pain in any part of the body or at multiple points, at any one time. This can occur at any time but the risk is likely to increase at later stages. The WHO (2007) offers a definition of the stages in HIV/AIDS infection (Table 9.2). The characteristics of these four stages indicate the possible causes of pain.

It is important, therefore, that pain management be more integrated into the total care of patients with HIV disease (Vogel et al., 1999). As in other

life-limiting conditions, establishing the cause of the pain or pains is a crucial element in the whole process and as can be seen from the range of diseases related to HIV/AIDS many investigative procedures may be necessary to establish the cause. These investigations in themselves will be a cause of pain as will the treatments prescribed. As Breitbart (2003) suggests the causes of pain in HIV/AIDS can be related to pain syndromes in patients, to the therapy they receive or to unrelated causes.

Activity 9.2

Review the three illustrative cases of life limiting diseases (cancer, MS and HIV/AIDS) discussed above.

How would you summarize the causes of pain in these conditions? In undertaking this activity think about categorizing the causes in such a way that will prove useful when considering other life-limiting conditions.

These three examples were offered as an illustration of the complexity of both life-limiting conditions and the way that pain may present as a symptom as part of the condition. You may have noticed when responding to Activity 9.2 that there were similar possible categories of causes of pain in the three examples. You may have categorized causes as ones related to:

- the condition itself;
- the complications associated with the condition;
- the treatment;
- unrelated conditions.

Having such a conceptual structure in mind can be helpful when assessing individuals in pain.

Key point

Pain in individuals with a life-limiting progressive condition may be caused by factors not related to that condition.

Pain assessment

Having explored the possible causes of pain in some life-limiting conditions, we now consider assessment of pain. As we highlighted in Chapter 4 good pain assessment is essential in the care and treatment of individuals. It is not our intention to repeat in this chapter content discussed in Chapter 4. Here we wish to highlight principles applicable to pain assessment in palliative care.

Nevertheless, it is important to re-emphasize here that in palliative care certain principles are central not only to the total care of individuals but also to the assessment of pain. These principles include the belief that we should care for individuals holistically and with respect to pain appreciate that it is multidimensional and the term *total pain* is consistent with this holistic approach. As a result when assessing pain we should consider the impact of the life-limiting condition on the individual from a physical, psychological, social and spiritual perspective as it is only then will we begin to have an understanding of the patient's unique and subjective pain experience (SIGN, 2008).

For some time the literature suggests that accurate management of pain and pain treatments rest on precise and ongoing assessment (De Wit et al., 1999; Livneh et al., 1998; Redmond, 1998; Rond et al., 1999).

Perhaps one of the most important issues that we should remember is that with life-limiting conditions the trajectory of the illness could vary over a long period of time resulting in the combination of acute and chronic pains from a variety of causes, some related to the condition and some not.

In Chapter 4 we examined the similarities and differences between acute and chronic pains. In the following activity we ask you to make a comparison between those types and palliative pain.

Activity 9.3

The following table contains characteristics of acute and chronic pain. Having considered these descriptions complete the column for palliative pain, highlighting any similarities or differences.

Acute pain	Chronic pain	Palliative pain
Recent onset	Pain which has lasted for long periods, generally more than six months, or persisting beyond the normal injury healing process	
Causal relationship: Injury Disease	May not always be an identifiable cause for the pain	
Possible to estimate length of duration	Duration of chronic pain unlimited – no idea of the timescale involved	

Acute pain	Chronic pain	Palliative pain
Recent onset	Pain which has lasted for long periods, generally more than six months, or persisting beyond the normal injury healing process	Varies depending on nature of the disease and response to therapies Usually but not always progressively worsens
Causal relationship: Injury Disease	May not always be an identifiable cause for the pain	Causal relationship normally due to disease but may be due to treatments
Possible to estimate length of duration	Duration of chronic pain unlimited – no idea of the timescale involved	Duration often unpredictable; may have a mixture of acute and chronic pains
		Limited by life expectancy resulting from underlying disease

During this activity your answer may have included similar points to those included in Table above. The important issue to take from the activity is that palliative pain may have some similarities to acute and chronic pain but equally needs to be considered as a specific and challenging type of pain in itself. This is because of the potential for a complex presentation where in any individual patient there may be incidents of only acute pain, at other times only chronic pain, but also a mixed pattern where both acute and chronic are present. The experience of pain is interpreted within an understanding that at least some of the pain experiences are a result of a condition that is limiting their life and individuals may be attributing all pain experience to the life-limiting condition. We as practitioners need to assess and reassess each situation without automatic attribution to the diagnosis.

As a result the focus of pain assessment may differ for each of the groups, based on the timescale and psychosocial factors involved.

Pain assessment tools in palliative care

Pain assessment tools can be a valuable aid to a health professional when assessing a patient's pain. Like all assessment tools, they can be used to form a baseline and means of evaluation. Each of the tools discussed in

Chapter 4 may have a place in the assessment of palliative pain. An important consideration is that the assessment of any individual's pain should be consistent and as a result the same tool or assessment process should be used so that a comparison can be made between assessments and pain events (SIGN, 2008). As a result no one assessment tool in itself has proved to be superior to another although unless consistent staff development occurs in a chosen tool's use the assessment will lack validity and reliability. In palliative pain, tools that only measure intensity will fail to be effective in the assessment process and therefore the tool adopted should facilitate an in-depth assessment.

Factors to consider during assessment

From your reading of this chapter and previous chapters in the book, you may have concluded that some of the following are important factors to consider in an assessment of palliative pain:

- the location or locations of the pain(s) experienced;
- the duration of each reported pain;
- the characteristics of each reported pain;
- the underlying cause of each pain if identifiable; for example, is the underlying cause related to treatments or investigations?

- the onset of each pain; for example, is it a new pain, one lasting for a few hours or days, or one that is chronic?
- if the pain is not new, then what care and treatment strategies have been prescribed?
- are there any exacerbating factors such as the time of day or mobility or lack of mobility?
- an objective observation of the pain.

Some of the assessment tools described in Chapter 4 help to capture this information, some do not. There is a balance required between sufficient depth without the assessment being so prolonged that it becomes difficult for both patient and practitioner.

Activity 9.4

Examine a pain assessment tool used in the practice of palliative care. Do you think it is *fit for purpose*? Try to be clear as to what it is about the tool that makes it appropriate or not.

Thomas (1997) felt that taking all the factors mentioned above into consideration could be a laborious process for the patient and nurse, although an ideal tool should provide data on these dimensions. Thomas (1997) advocated the use of the McGill Pain Questionnaire (MPQ) and the brief pain inventory (BPI); the BPI being developed for clinical use with patients too ill to be subjected to long exhausting assessment tools. Thomas also advocated the use of the Memorial Pain Assessment Card (MPAC) (Fishman et al., 1987). It is clear from Thomas's suggestions that there may not be the ideal assessment tool for all situations and patients. Indeed, the health professional and any individual patient may benefit from a different assessment tool at different stages of their life-limiting condition; for example, when level of consciousness fluctuates or cognitive ability deteriorates. This can certainly be a main factor with many life-limiting illnesses. According to Schofield et al. (2008) there are many behavioural pain scales that have been developed, such as Abbey et al. (2004), and include several important factors such as physiological observations, facial expressions, body movements, verbalizations, changes in interpersonal interactions,

changes in activity or routines and changes in mental status.

The assessment so far has emphasized a measurement of the physical dimension of the pain experience. To more accurately understand the patient's experience, we too must appreciate the psychosocial and spiritual dimensions. As a result it is important to consider factors that may influence the patient's experience of pain.

Psychosocial factors influencing the pain experience

Psychosocial aspects of painful conditions play a major role in the manner in which patients will tolerate, describe and cope with their pain. Understanding these influences are important for all chronic pains, not just for those originating from a life-limiting condition.

Some of the psychological factors affecting pain responses may be:

1. Cultural differences
2. Observational learning (modelling)
3. Cognitive appraisal
4. Fear and anxiety
5. Neuroticism and extroversion
6. Perceived control of events
7. Coping style

(Cousins, 1994: 367)

1. *Cultural differences:* the cultural differences between individuals, often learnt through primary socialization, have been found to influence expressions of pain. Sternbach and Tursky (1965) found that women from different cultures had a uniform sensation threshold but different tolerance levels. Most culture differences are enforced through upbringing; old Americans are known for their restraint regarding public shows of emotion, whereas Italians, for example, are known for their passion and public vociferation. From your own experiences you may have come across such differences. No attitude is right or wrong. As carers, however, we must be aware of our own values and beliefs and ensure we do not impose them on those we care for. As we have all heard many times: *'Pain is whatever the experiencing person says it is and exists*

whenever he says it does' (McCaffery and Beebe, 1999: 16).

(2) *Observational learning:* this includes behaviour learnt from childhood and past experiences of pain. Childhood experiences often influence in later life the way we express, or do not express our emotions. As a child I was often told to 'rub it better' and was encouraged to do something else to 'take your mind off it'. This attitude is one I have kept and indeed passed on to my own children. Some children, on the other hand, are cuddled and given treats if they are injured, and can often feign injury for the rewards it produces. In a small number of patients with chronic pain, the rewards that being in pain can produce are so beneficial that any attempts to improve the situation for the patient fails. These rewards can be financial, as in state benefits, or personal with family members; for example, undertake all household chores.

Past experiences with health care professionals and pain management will also affect the patient's pain. The chronic pain patient that has had their pain disregarded by specialists as there was no identified organic cause for the pain will often be angry and frustrated. Before pain assessment can be undertaken, it is important to discuss the history of the pain and dispel fears concerning this. It is important to emphasize that it is possible for pain to exist even in the absence of any obvious organic cause.

(3) *Cognitive appraisal:* The meaning of the pain to the patient will affect their expression of the pain. Elderly patients will often put up with the pain of arthritis as part of 'getting older'. Patients with pain due to a life-limiting illness can be more anxious and often angry. Patients with chronic non-malignant pain can often become depressed, as no end to the pain is apparent. It is important then to remember the context in which the patient is experiencing the pain and the perceived course of the condition.

(4) *Fear and anxiety:* fear and anxiety are as difficult to define as pain. Circumstances associated with pain are some of the most potent in aggravating such fears. The anxiety experienced by other family members is often transferred directly to the patient and we have all witnessed the patient

who becomes more distressed as the result of a visit by family members. Boyle and Parbrook (1977) concluded that the experience of pain is most often heightened in those with anxious personalities, thus pointing out the importance of effective patient communication and counselling.

(5) *Neuroticism, introversion and extroversion:* neuroticism refers to a person's emotional stability, and is often linked to trait anxiety levels. Many discussions have arisen over the effects of neuroticism on pain experiences. Some patients with high anxiety or neurotic tendencies can be inclined to exaggerate pain expressions.

Those with more introverted personalities may find it more difficult to express their pain while extroverts are generally believed to complain more of pain, and studies have shown a link between extroversion and analgesia scores. Bond (1979) said that assessing personality gives an indication as to how individuals usually respond to fears and anxieties in their lives, and has identified lower pain thresholds in those individuals classed as introverts. It becomes apparent then that personality tendencies can influence the patient's experience of pain, and is a factor carers must be aware of.

(6) *Perceived control of events:* the concept of control can be considered on a continuum between external control, in which the surrounding environment affects the individual and is responsible for controlling, or not, the pain, and internal control, where events are due to the actions of the individual. When in pain, patients feel that they have to convince carers of the reality of their pain in order to receive treatment. In chronic pain, patients often feel that the pain controls their lives. One of the strategies for chronic pain management is to return the **locus of control** to the patient, in order that they have the 'tools' to control the pain. This has an effect on the mental state of the individual and helps in alleviating depression, which is a common feature in chronic non-malignant pain patients.

(7) *Coping style:* how patients cope with their pain depends largely on their emotional state and how they visualize their situation. Copp (1994) described five roles a patient may assume.

- The '**victim**' sees pain as all-powerful and relies on the carer to relieve that pain. Becoming reliant on others causes a loss of self-control. Loss of independence and control is a precursor to depression.
- The '**soldier**' finds the experience of pain a test, and themselves a fighter who will confront the pain. The patient with this psychological attribute may, initially, be seen to cope with the pain well, but as time goes on, the chronic pain patient may become depressed due to the unrelenting nature of the pain experience.
- The '*seer/thinker*' dwells on *why* questions. Crisson and Keefe (1988) stated that patients with this psychological trait tend to use maladaptive coping mechanisms that increase the perception of pain and leaves the patient vulnerable to depression.
- The 'watcher/waiter' awaits pain that may invade them at any time. These patients cope by anticipating pain and looking for early warning signs. They may appear to be totally enveloped in their pain.
- The 'consumer' expects the carer to stand by and provide promised pain relief, and copes with bonding through them. Depending on the values, attitudes and beliefs of the carer, this coping mechanism may be effective, but as we found when discussing the social relationship of depression and chronic pain, this may also serve to increase both the experience of chronic pain and depression, if support is lacking.

Unfortunately, we are aware that people do not conveniently adopt an individual coping strategy, but can adopt or demonstrate more than one. Nevertheless, an understanding of such strategies is useful in both the assessment and management of palliative pain as it offers possible explanations for the patient's response and involvement.

Consequences of pain

The consequences of pain inevitably impact on the physical, psychosocial and spiritual dimensions of individuals and these consequences should be considered in both pain assessment and management.

Activity 9.5

Read the following case study and consider the consequences of Dennis's pain from a physical, psychological, social and spiritual perspective.

Dennis is a 55-year-old painter and decorator who is self-employed. Dennis has not paid national insurance contributions for years, as he saw no point. He is married to Diane and they have two sons aged 18 and 21. Both boys live at home in their small three-bedroomed council house. Dennis enjoys a drink every day in the local pub most evenings, while Diane enjoys her bingo. Diane works at the local school as a cleaner and a dinner lady, working long split hours. They both smoke heavily.

Dennis has visited his general practitioner with increasing shortness of breath; he has no cough, no wheeze, and no other specific symptoms, other than an ache and a slight 'hunch' in his posture. His GP decides to send Dennis for a chest X-ray. Following the X-ray Dennis is referred to the chest physician for a further consultation, where he is diagnosed with mesothelioma, a form of cancer.

Within the following few months Dennis suffered with increasing symptoms, his pain became steadily worse, mainly pain on breathing over the rib area; it is worse on movement. Walking up and down stairs are a problem and Dennis has only one toilet which is downstairs. He has one living room, so is currently sleeping on the sofa, as it is too painful to complete the stairs.

He is now not able to continue working and finances have become a problem. They are relying on Diane's wage, who is also finding work a problem due to the increasing care needs at home.

Dennis is only able to go to the pub

when he can get a lift, as he cannot manage to walk the short distance.

What are the consequences of Dennis's pain?

Physical:

Psychological:

Social:

Spiritual:

When we look at the information that we are given, as small as it may appear, we can gain a great deal of information regarding Dennis and the potential consequences that pain can have on his life.

Physical

The increasing pain in Dennis's chest is having a direct effect on his breathing. Dennis is trying to compensate for the pain and is also developing a slight hunch where he is sitting in an awkward position. Dennis is finding mobility more difficult due to the increased pain. This is having a direct effect on the other three components.

Psychological

Dennis may associate his increasing pain with deterioration of his disease and it is also a constant reminder of his illness. We see Dennis is less able to go out and to work, therefore it can have a direct effect on his mood with increasing feelings of depression and sadness.

Social

This can be directly linked to the above two categories, as there can be a direct effect on Dennis's ability to move around the house and also to have a direct effect on his social life. This in turn can enhance feelings of

lack of control while increasing the feelings of isolation. Dennis having been his own boss for many years has not relied on anyone and his social circle is separate from that of his family; it could therefore aid feelings of resentment.

Spiritual

This can be an overview of all the previous three; it can also be linked to what Dennis's perception is of his future. This is intrinsically linked to hope and the 'why me?' questions that can arise. With the diagnosis of a life-limiting disease perceptions of hope may fluctuate; what is hoped for initially may be for the diagnosis to be wrong and/or for a cure to be found. This can change to hope for treatments to work, to slow things down, or to ease pain. It is essential that hope is obtainable, or at least not unattainable, as this can be a factor in losing hope. What factors affect the loss of hope are again very individual, unrealistic goals, loss of control, increasing symptoms, raised fear could all affect what hope you may have had.

Discussing hope and living with the diagnosis of a life-limiting disease in the same sentence can appear arduous. However, the discussion of hope can be seen as an essential part of holistic care. As a result, when considering the assessment of the pain experience, we should consider pain's impact on the individual.

Barriers to pain assessment and management

Having considered assessment, factors that may influence that process and the consequences of the pain experience, we also need to be aware of our own attitudes and feelings and how these can influence and potentially form barriers when looking at a patient's perception, description of pain and management of that experience.

There are a number of potential barriers to pain assessment exhibited by health professionals. Some of these are more easily remedied than others and some are a result of our inability to perceive the situation accurately. More easily remedied barriers include:

- a lack of education concerning the specific life-limiting condition of the patient;
- the assessment tools in use;

- the factors that influence perception or consequences of the condition.

There are also barriers related to working practices. For example:

- poor assessment as result of time pressures;
- care occurring in inappropriate clinical areas or;
- insufficient staff of appropriate experience.

Barriers can occur because of our own perception of events or attitudes towards the pain experience of others. This can be as a result of the patient's own attitudes or behaviour; for example, denial of disease, or reluctance to report pain, but can also occur as a result of our own values, beliefs and attitudes concerning the nature of pain and how it should be expressed. This in turn may be influenced by our own pain experiences from both a personal and professional perspective. As a result we interpret events from our own perspective rather than that of the individual experiencing pain.

When assessing pain we should also consider:

- What influencing factors could be impacting on the patient's assessment of pain?
- What are the consequences of the pain experience on the individual?
- What potential barriers am I bringing to the assessment?

Key point

Pain assessment should consider the impact of the life-limiting condition on the individual from a physical, psychological, social and spiritual perspective; and consider factors that influence the assessment and the barriers to assessment. It is only then will we begin to have an understanding of the patient's unique and subjective pain experience.

Pharmacological and non-pharmacological management of pain in palliative care

We have focused on three life-limiting conditions to illustrate how pain may manifest itself in palliative care. We have also been careful to emphasize the individual nature of pain, its causes and consequences. As a result practitioners have to develop care plans that are specific to the needs of individuals based on their understanding of the life-limiting condition and how it impacts on the pain experience. It is not possible to offer a detailed discussion on the management of pain in all life-limiting conditions in a chapter of this size and so we have included a list of suggested readings at the end of the chapter. We are also being selective in terms of the management strategies discussed. Earlier we identified the causes of pain and suggested they could be associated with:

- the condition itself;
- the complications associated with the condition;
- the treatment;
- unrelated conditions.

We need to bear these causes in mind when considering an appropriate plan of care. Here, we focus on pain experienced in cancer, recognizing the limitation of doing so but also appreciating that pain management in palliative settings is still very much associated with this diagnostic group. Hopefully, this is changing as health providers appreciate the need for palliative services in a much wider range of life-limiting conditions. The principles we discuss here are often useful in other life-limiting conditions. Underpinning this treatment is the information gained during assessment and evaluation.

Approaches to pain management in patients who have cancer

The WHO (1996) suggest six broad approaches to the management of pain (Fig. 9.3).

Clearly, the management strategy utilized will depend on an effective assessment. This will dictate which of the approaches is best suited at any one time or in any particular combination. What will be certain is that the approaches will differ over time as the condition progresses and the needs of the individual changes.

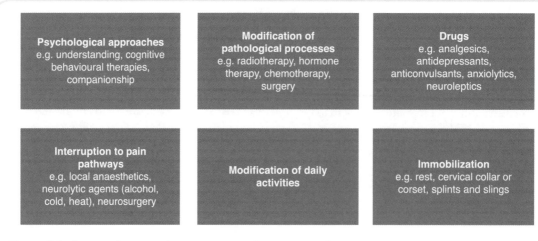

Psychological approaches e.g. understanding, cognitive behavioural therapies, companionship	**Modification of pathological processes** e.g. radiotherapy, hormone therapy, chemotherapy, surgery	**Drugs** e.g. analgesics, antidepressants, anticonvulsants, anxiolytics, neuroleptics
Interruption to pain pathways e.g. local anaesthetics, neurolytic agents (alcohol, cold, heat), neurosurgery	**Modification of daily activities**	**Immobilization** e.g. rest, cervical collar or corset, splints and slings

Figure 9.3 Approaches to pain management in cancer patients
Source: adopted from WHO (1996)

Drug management

Before we look at specific drugs and drug regimens, it is useful to remind ourselves that drugs in themselves may not be successful in managing the individual's pain. Even when they are the most apt choice there are numerous reasons for why they may not be effective. Some of these reasons are a result of health professional attitudes and practices. As Twycross and Wilcock (2001) remind us, there are numerous potential bad practices that impact on the effectiveness of the prescribed drug:

- inability to distinguish between pains caused by cancer and pain that is related to another cause;
- failure to evaluate each individual pain and treat accordingly;
- failure to use non-drug measures, especially in muscle spasm pain;
- failure to use NSAID and opioids in combination;
- failure to use adjuvant analgesics especially anti-depressants and anti-epileptics;
- a *laissez-faire* attitude to drug times and to education of patient and family;
- changing to an alternative analgesic before optimizing the dose and timing of the previous analgesic;
- combining analgesics inappropriately;
- failure to appreciate that a mixed agonist-

antagonist should not be used in conjunction with codeine and morphine;
- reluctance to prescribe morphine;
- changing from a strong opioid to an inadequate dose of morphine;
- reducing the interval between administrations instead of increasing the dose;
- using injections when oral medication is possible;
- failure to monitor and control adverse effects of medication, especially constipation;
- lack of attention to psychosocial issues;
- failure to listen to the patient.

(Twycross and Wilcock, 2002: 28)

Even so, the mainstay of pain management is drug therapy. The WHO guidelines on cancer pain, symptom control and palliative care recommend that doctors and other health professionals know how to use just a few drugs well. The basic drug list recommended by WHO since the publication of the first cancer pain relief guidelines in 1986 includes non-opioids, weak opioids, strong opioids and adjuvants. They suggest that drugs should be given:

- by mouth;
- by the clock;
- in a dose optimal to the patient.

In combination with the 'analgesic ladder' (Fig. 9.4) this guidance offers simple and sequential advice.

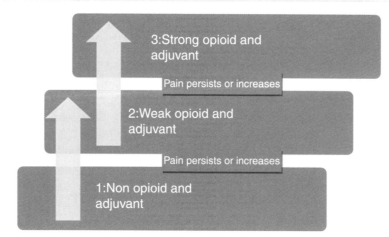

Figure 9.4 WHO (1986) analgesic ladder

The analgesic ladder

Pain should be controlled with oral therapy when possible. Rectal or subcutaneous infusions are alternatives in those patients who have difficulty in swallowing or when there is uncontrolled vomiting.

Constant pain requires regular therapy, therefore analgesia should be given by the clock with the next dose given before the previous one wears off. It may be necessary for a patient to need analgesia in between each dose. This breakthrough analgesia should be available at 50–100 per cent of the four-hourly dose. The choice of analgesia depends on the severity of pain and previous analgesia, not on the stage of the disease. Morphine is the drug of choice; other opioids are used only if there are specific indications.

There are no standard doses for opioid drugs. The correct dose is that which relieves the pain. The only drugs that have limits are those on step one and two, which have maximum dosages to follow. Patients should be titrated with immediate release morphine, which is converted to controlled release when appropriate. The adverse effects of opiods should be anticipated and treated and immediate release morphine should be available for breakthrough pain. It is essential that other pains such as neuropathic and bone pain should be treated accordingly. It is wise for the individual patient to work out their own regime. However, dosages can be linked to specific

times such as breakfast/wake up or bedtime. Patients should be advised to keep a diary of the dosages they take and exactly when they take them. As SIGN (2008) guidelines remind us, the development of new opioids, delivery routes and widespread availability create more choice for the practitioner than was available at the development of the WHO ladder (Fig. 9.4).

A thorough patient assessment will ensure that severity, type and cause of pain are considered when considering management. The WHO analgesic ladder depends on such an assessment as the severity of the pain will determine the strength of analgesic, and the cause and type of pain, the choice of adjuvant therapy. As a result a consistency in pain rating is important when utilizing the analgesic ladder. The SIGN (2008), drawing on a limited evidence, is confident in their transference of patient's pain scores to analgesic ladder category (Table 9.3).

These guidelines produce effective control of chronic cancer pain in about 80 per cent of patients. In the remaining 20 per cent other methods of pain control must be considered, including spinal administration of opioid analgesics alone or in combination with local anaesthetics or other drugs (WHO, 1986).

Although devised for use in cancer care the principles of this approach to pain management has found support in other areas of palliative care. For example, Breitbart (2003) looked at the guidelines for the

WHO analgesic ladder step	Score on numerical rating scale	Analgesic choice
1 (mild pain)	< 3 out of 10	Paracetamol and NSAIDs
2 (mild to moderate pain)	3–6 out of 10	Weak opioids (e.g. codeine) plus paracetamol and NSAIDs
3 (severe pain)	> 6 out of 10	Strong opioid (e.g. morphine)

Table 9.3 Relationship between WHO analgesic ladder steps and numerical rating scale score
Source: Adapted from SIGN (2008)

management of HIV/AIDS pain suggesting that clinicians feel comfortable using the ladder and the accompanying principles.

Adjuvant drugs are very valuable in the management of pain, and can be used in conjunction with non-opioids and opioids, or used as stand alone treatments. We had some discussion of their use in Chapter 5. Here their use in palliative care is summarized in Table 9.4.

Modification of pathological processes

Radiotherapy

Over 50 per cent of cancer patients will receive radiotherapy (Hoskin and Makin, 1998) either as a stand-alone treatment or in combination with another. The disruption that radiotherapy can bring to a patient can be difficult to describe, as often this can mean a daily journey to and from the hospital.

Information and communication is essential for patients to understand what to expect prior to and during treatment. Radiotherapy can be a long process for the cancer patient. However, as a treatment for cancer pain, such as bone metastases, often few visits are required and the duration of each is shorter. The objective with radiotherapy as pain relief is simple: to relieve the pain and promote optimal quality of life for the patient; it is one of the most effective remedies for bone pain. One systematic review carried out in 1999 (McQuay et al., 1999) demonstrated complete relief at one month in 27 per cent of patients. In another 42 per cent of patients there was at least 50 per cent relief from pain.

Chemotherapy

Literally this means drug treatment; in practice, the term 'chemotherapy' is used to describe the treatment given using cytotoxic drugs. The aim of chemotherapy treatment can also vary. In the treatment of pain the aim is to potentially shrink the tumour, or reduce the growth rate, therefore relieving the painful symptom. However, it can result in troublesome side-effects.

Surgery

This is often a reasonable option in some cases. Treatment decisions are based on many different factors. It is imperative that the health professionals understand these so they can convey them to the patient, who often needs an explanation as to why they are or are not having certain treatment. Orthopaedic surgery is a good example for the relief of pain, such as from spinal metastases and pathological fractures.

Endocrine therapy

A number of cancers depend on a hormonal environment in which to develop; breast and prostate being the most common. This therapy is not associated with curative treatment, but with disease regression, and symptom management. It is often used as an adjuvant treatment.

Interruption to pain pathways

Local anaesthetics

These act by reversibly blocking peripheral nerve impulses. They affect autonomic, sensory (pain temperature, touch and pressure) and motor fibres

Adjuvant drug	Use	Note
Anticonvulsants (e.g. gabapentin; carbamazepine)	Neuropathic pain	Until recently there has been no drug of choice but carbamazepine and sodium valproate are commonly used. However, in the elderly, anticonvulsant drugs used in relatively high doses can produce sedation and dizziness. Gabapentin has been shown to be efficacious in neuropathic pain even in these vulnerable groups
Antidepressants (e.g. amitriptyline; imipramine)	Neuropathic pain	As with the antidepressant action of these drugs, it takes 7–10 days after treatment before any therapeutic effect becomes noticeable. A mild but very uncomfortable side-effect in palliative patients is a dry mouth. Thirteen per cent of patients in one systematic review had to withdraw because of side-effects (Saarto and Wiffen, 2007)
Corticosteriods	Bone and nerve root pain	
Antispasmodics	Colic	
Muscle relaxants	Severe muscle spasm	
Lignocaine 5% plaster	Posthepatic neuralgia	Superior to placebo (Galer et al., 2002; Binder et al., 2009). Binder et al. noted drug-related adverse events in 13.6% of the sample
Anaesthetic drugs (e.g. ketamine)	Persistent, uncontrolled pain Used in neuropathic, ischaemic limb, and refractory pain in cancer. Less effective in long-standing neuropathic pain	Administered along with a strong opioid; current practice is to reduce opioid dose when ketamine started Needs close supervision when used

Table 9.4 Examples of adjuvant drugs used in palliative care

depending on the drug and concentration used and where they are placed. Local anaesthetics are used to infiltrate wounds during surgery as well as in epidural analgesia solutions but are short-acting drugs. Drug regimes should be kept as simple as practically possible while ensuring that the pain experience is as controlled as practically possible.

Non-pharmocological treatment: psychological and physical approaches

Cognitive behavioural therapy (CBT)

CBT is a short- to medium-term therapy that focuses on thoughts and behaviour. The CBT therapist can help the patient to study their beliefs, insights and identify how these can impact on their emotional welfare, and actions. So in the relationship pain, patients are taught skills that can help them cope with the pain. It is imperative that this is structured to the patient's own set of goals and is truly subjective (Paz and Seymour, 2004). There is strong evidence to support its use in the management of chronic non-malignant pain (Morley et al., 1999) and in improving quality of life in patients with cancer (Graves, 2003).

Complementary therapies

Meditation relaxation and guided imagery

Basic meditation can often be started by learning some basic techniques. Cicala (2001) suggests this can be helpful to learn, allowing the patient to remain calm and also relaxed. Relaxation is very similar; pre-recorded relaxation tapes are easily available; often assisting the patient to identify what they find relaxes them can be a useful process. Guided imagery is one such type of relaxation; this focuses on an image or a place, which can be real or completely imaginary, where they feel safe and therefore calm.

Acupuncture

According to Beech (2001) this is one of the most widely researched complementary therapies, frequently being used to assist with the management of pain. Acupuncture has been used to treat acute post-operative pain in cancer patients and also chronic or intractable pain associated with the cancer or its various treatments; Woollam and Jackson (1998) suggest acupuncture is currently used in over 84 per cent of pain clinics. When used in cancer pain there seems to be some conflicting evidence of its efficacy. Alimi et al. (2003), using auricular acupuncture, showed a decrease in pain in 36 per cent in two months compared with a 2 per cent decrease in the placebo group while one systematic review of seven relevant studies (Lee et al., 2005) concluded that there was no evidence to support its use.

Transcutaneous electrical nerve stimulation (TENS)

This applies a controlled low voltage electric current through electrodes placed on the skin. The waveform of the machine stimulates and interferes with the transmission of messages via nerve fibres, 70 per cent of patients responding initially with pain relief (Forbes and Faull, 1998). It is often trial and error by the patient using the machine to find the most effective usage, or type of shock used.

Massage, aromatherapy, reflexology

One of the earliest senses we develop is touch. If it hurts it is natural to rub it. Massage is a generic term for techniques that involve touching, pressing, kneading soft tissue for therapeutic purpose. It is the basis for reflexology and aromatherapy but can be therapeutic in its own right. Aromatherapy is the therapeutic use of specifically prepared plant essential oils which are found in flowers, leaves, seeds, wood, root and bark. Essential oils are applied in a variety of ways, which include massage, vaporisers, baths, creams and lotions, and compresses, and are absorbed through the skin, diluted in carrier oil or by inhalation. Massage is the most widely used medium for applying essentials oils. Reflexology is also known as zone therapy; it is a massage technique that concentrates on the feet. Specific areas of the feet are representational to certain organs and areas of the body. The systematic application of pressure, using the thumb and fingers, to specific reflex points on the feet either offers the therapist information regarding the organ or can lead to a therapeutic change, such as reduction in pain. Although some studies (Post-White et al., 2003; Soden et al., 2004) suggest massage and aromatherapy have some short-term benefits on well-being, there was conflicting evidence as to their benefits in longer-term pain relief. The impact of reflexology on pain is poorly researched. One randomized controlled trial (RCT) (Stephenson et al., 2007) identified a reduction in pain in 34 per cent compared to a 2 per cent reduction in the control group.

Immobilization

There are circumstances where immobilization would seem a sensible approach; for example, following a pathological fracture where stabilization of the fracture using e.g. plaster of Paris, will help reduce pain. Professional opinion has changed significantly over the years concerning immobilization in certain chronic pains; for example, low back pain. Twenty-five years ago the treatment for low back pain could have included the use of pethidine, valium and pelvic traction while now, for a similar degree of pain and disability, the individual would be encouraged to mobilize and take a co-analgesic.

Rehabilitation – modification of daily activities

A rehabilitative approach can help people with advancing, life-threatening disease lead satisfying lives within the restrictions of their illness; and this approach can be a vital part of palliative care.

> *Encouragement, support and help is provided to help patients achieve their potential, and maintain their independence for as long as possible, regardless of life expectancy. It is about quality of living, while at the same time preparing for dying ... rehabilitation should be considered a fundamental part of all palliative care services, wherever they are based.*
>
> (NCPC, 2000: 3)

The guidance from NICE (2004) supports this approach to care relevant to all palliative care services.

Referral to other members of the multi-professional team can offer an invaluable role in the management and modification of day-to-day living. This can include identifying triggers and then reviewing the daily routine to find ways to build up energy and conserve it. Encouraging individuals to be realistic about activity can be useful although these lifestyle adjustments can be challenging. It can be useful to get the patient to complete a diary, detailing all activities, as this can help to form a picture of which activities of living are proving problematic.

Key point

A range of pharmacological and non-pharmacological approaches are likely to be needed in the management of pain in palliative conditions.

Summary

In this chapter you have explored the meaning of palliative care and the assessment and management of pain in a range of life-limiting conditions. This approach has highlighted the need for a detailed assessment and exploration of the many potential causes of the pain experience. This approach has also illustrated the differences in the pain experience in different medical diagnoses, highlighting the importance of individualized care. A number of care strategies have been explored. Although those strategies are ones considered pertinent for the management of cancer pain, we have asked you to consider their applicability in other life-limiting conditions. As a result you should be able to:

- define the key concepts of palliative care;
- identify the possible causes of pain in three life-limiting conditions;
- consider the role of assessment and the appropriateness of using pain assessment tools in the management of life-limiting conditions;
- suggest a range of pharmacological and non-pharmacological approaches to pain management.

In addition, following completion of the reflective activity below, consider the content of this chapter as a basis for the care of patients with a life-limiting condition within your area of practice.

Reflective activity

As a conclusion to this chapter, consider how knowledge of this theory will help you in your future practice. Try to be specific and use the following points/questions as a guide.

- *State* which elements of the chapter will help you in your future practice.
- *Elaborate:* be specific in terms of how this knowledge and understanding can be used in practice.
- *Give examples:* of care events which would benefit from what you have learnt.
- What are the *implications* if you change the way you practise.

You may prefer to use a reflective model such as Gibbs's (1988) to guide your reflection (see Appendix at the end of this book).

Think of a specific example as the starting point. This may have been a specific example from clinical practice or from your own or family's experiences of palliative care. The intent of this reflection would be to evaluate your present practice in light of your greater understanding of pain management in palliative care. Although we have offered specific life-limiting conditions to illustrate the discussion, you may like to focus on a different client group as a means of transferring your knowledge into a new area of care.

Consider:

- how well the pain was assessed;
- if all causes of pain were identified;
- what approaches to pain management were adopted.

References

Abbey, J., Piller, N., De Bellis, A. et al. (2004) The Abbey pain scale: a 1-minute numerical indicator for people with end-stage dementia, *International Journal Palliative Nursing*, 10(1): 6–13.

Alimi, D., Rubino, C., Pichard-Leandri, E., Fermand-Brule, S., Dubreuil-Lemaire, M. and Hill, C. (2003) Analgesic effect of auricular acupuncture for cancer pain: a randomized, blinded, controlled trial, *Journal of Clinical Oncology*, 21(22): 4120–6.

Archibald, C.J. et al. (1994) Pain prevalence, severity and impact in a clinic sample of multiple sclerosis patients, *Pain*, 58(1): 89–93.

AVERT (2009) Pain in people with HIV. Available online at www.avert.org/aids-pain.htm. (accessed 16 September 2009).

Beech, N. (2001) Complementary therapies in J. Corner and C. Bailey (2001) *Cancer Nursing Care in Context*. Oxford: Blackwell Science.

Binder, A., Bruxelle, J., Rogers, P., Hans, G., Bösl, I., and Baron, R. (2009) Topical 5% lidocaine (lignocaine) medicated plaster treatment for post-herpetic neuralgia: results of a double-blind, placebo-controlled, multinational efficacy and safety trial, *Clinical Drug Investigation*, 29(6): 393–408.

Bond, M. (1979) *Pain: Its Nature Analysis and Treatment*. London: Churchill Livingstone.

Boyle, P. and Parbrook, G.D. (1977) The inter relationship of personality and post operative analgesia, *British Journal of Anaesthesia*, 49: 259–63.

Breitbart, W. (2003) Pain, in J.F. O'Neill, P.A. Selwyn and H. Schietinger (eds) *The Clinical Guide to Supportive and Palliative Care for HIV/AIDS*. Rockville, M.D: Health Resources and Services Administration. Available online at www.hab.hrsg.gov/tools/palliative (accessed 22 June 2010).

Cancer Research UK (2009) *UK cancer mortality statistics*. London: Cancer Research UK. Available online at www.info.cancerresearchuk.org/cancerstats/mortality/?a= 5441 (accessed 27 July 2009).

Cicala, R.S. (ed.) (2001) *The Cancer Pain Sourcebook*. Lincolnwood, IL: Contemporary Books.

Copp, L.A. (1994) Pain assessment, management and research: the nurse's role, in H.B. Gibson (ed.) *Psychology, Pain and Anaesthesia*. London: Chapman & Hall.

Cousins, M. (1964) Acute post operative pain, in R. Melzack and P.D. Wall (eds) *The Textbook of Pain*. London: Churchill Livingstone.

Crisson J.E. and Keefe F.J. (1988) The relationship of locus of control to pain coping strategies and psychological distress in chronic pain patients, *Pain*, 35: 147–54.

De wit, R., Van Dam, F., Vielvoye-kerkmeer, A., Malten, C. and Abu-Saad, H.H. (1999) The treatment of chronic pain in a cancer hospital in the Netherlands, *Journal of Pain and Symptom Management*, 17(5): 333–50.

Faull, C. and Woof, R. (2002) *Palliative Care: An Oxford Core Text*. Maidenhead: Oxford University Press.

Fishman, B., Pasternak, S., Wallenstein, S.L., Houde, R.W., Holland, J.C. and Foley, K.M. (1987) The memorial pain assessment card: a valid instrument for the evaluation of cancer pain, *Cancer*, 60: 1151–80.

Forbes, K. and Faull, C. (1998) The principles of pain management in C. Faull, Y. Carter and R. Woof (eds) *Handbook of Palliative Care*. Oxford: Blackwell Science.

Galer, B., Jensen, M., Ma, T., Davies, P. and Rowbotham, M. (2002) The lidocaine patch 5% effectively treats all neuropathic pain qualities: results of a randomised double blind vehicle-controlled, 3 week efficacy study with the use of the neuropathic pain scale, *Clinical Journal of Pain*, 18(5): 297–301.

Gibbs, G. (1988) *Learning by Doing: A Guide to Teaching and Learning Methods*. Oxford: Further Education Unit, Oxford Polytechnic.

Gold Standards Framework (GSF) (2006) Available online at www.goldstandardsframework.nhs.uk (accessed August 2009).

Graves, K.D. (2003) Social cognitive theory and cancer patients' quality of life: a meta-analysis of psychosocial intervention components, *Health Psychology*, 22(2): 210–19.

Hoskin, P. and Makin, W. (1998) *Oncology for Palliative Medicine*. Oxford: Oxford University Press.

Kaye, P. (1999) *Decision Making in Palliative Care*. Northampton: EPL Publications.

Lee, H., Schmidt, K. and Ernst, E. (2005) Acupuncture for the relief of cancer related pain: a systematic review, *European Journal of Pain*, 9(4): 437–44.

Livneh, J., Garber, A. and Shaevich, E. (1998) Assessment and documentation of pain in oncology patients, *International Journal of Palliative Nursing*, 4(4): 169–75.

McQuay, H.J., Collins, S., Carroll, D. and Moore, R.A. (1999) *Radiotherapy for the Palliation of Painful Bone Metastases* (Cochrane Review). Chichester: Wiley. Available online at www.mrw.interscience.wiley.com/cochrane/clsysrev/articles/CD001793/pdf_fs.html (accessed 18 September 2009).

McCaffery, M. and Beebe, A. (1999) *Pain: Clinical Manual*, 2nd edn. St Louis, MI: C V Mosby

Morley, S. Eccleston, C. and Williams, A. (1999) A systematic review and meta analysis of randomised controlled trials of cognitive behaviour therapy and behaviour therapy for chronic pain in adults, excluding headache, *Pain*, 80(1–2): 1–13.

Multiple Sclerosis Society (2009) *About Us*. Available online at www.mssociety.org.uk/about_ms/index.html (accessed 22 June 2010).

Murray, S.A., Kendall, M., Boyd, K. and Sheikh, A. (2005) Illness trajectories and palliative care, *British Medical Journal*, 330: 1007–11.

National Council for Palliative Care (NCPC) (2000) *Fulfilling Lives Rehabilitation in Palliative Care*. Available online at www.ncpc.org.uk.

National Council of Hospice and Specialist Palliative Care Services (NCHSPCS) (1995) *Specialist Palliative Care: A Statement of Definitions*. London: NCHSPCS.

National Institute for Clinical Excellence (NICE) (2004) *Improving Supportive and Palliative Care for Adults with Cancer*. London: NICE.

Payne, S., Sheldon, F., Jarrett, N., Large, S., Smith, P., Davis, C.L., Turner, P. and George, S. (2002) Differences in understandings of specialist palliative care amongst service providers and commissioners in South London, *Palliative Medicine*, 16: 395–402.

Paz, S. and Seymour, J. (2004) Working with difficult symptoms, in S. Payne, J. Seymour, and C. Ingleton (eds) *Palliative Care Nursing: Principles and Evidence for Practice*. Maidenhead: Open University Press.

Plumb, S. (2006) *MS and Palliative Care: A Guide for Health and Social Care Professionals*. London: Multiple Sclerosis Society.

Post-White, J., Kinney, M., Savik, K., Gau, J. and Wilcox, C.I.L. (2003) Therapeutic massage and healing touch improve symptoms in cancer, *Integrated Cancer Therapy*, 2(4): 332–44.

Redmond, K. (1998) Barriers to the effective management of pain, *International Journal of Palliative Nursing*, 4(6): 276–83.

Rond, M.E., DeWit, R. and De Dam (1999) Daily pain assessment: value for nurses and patients, *Journal of Advanced Nursing*, 29(2): 436–44.

Saarto, T. and Wiffen, P. (2007) *Antidepressants for Neuropathic Pain* (Cochrane Database of Systematic Review). Chichester: Wiley. Available online at www.mrw.interscience.wiley.com/cochrane/clsysrev/articles/CD005454/frame.html (accessed 18 September 2009).

Scottish Intercollegiate Guidelines Network (SIGN) (2008) *Control of Pain in Adults with Cancer: A National Clinical Guideline*. Edinburgh: NHS.

Soden, K., Vincent, K., Craske, S., Lucas, C. and Ashley, S. (2004) A randomized controlled trial of aromatherapy massage in a hospice setting, *Palliative Medicine*, 18(2): 87–92.

Schofield, P., O'Mahony, S., Collett, B. and Potter J. (2008) Guidance for the assessment of pain in older adults: a literature review, *British Journal of Nursing*, 17(14): 914–18.

Stephenson, N.L.N., Melvin Swanson, M., Dalton, J., Keefe, F.J. and Engelke, M. (2007) Partner-delivered reflexology: effects on cancer pain and anxiety, *Oncology Nursing Forum*, 34(1): 127–32.

Sternbach, R.A. and Tursky (1965) Ethnic differences among housewives in psychophysical and skin potential to electric shock, *Psychophysiology*, 1(3): 241–6.

Thomas, V.N. (1997) (ed.) *Pain: Its Nature and Management*. London: Bailliere Tindall.

Twycross, R. and Wilcock, A. (2001) *Symptom Management in Advanced Cancer*, 3rd edn. Abingdon: Radcliffe Medical Press.

Vogel, D., Rosenfeld, B., Breitbart, W. et al. (1999) Symptom prevalence, characteristics, and distress in AIDS outpatients, *Journal of Pain Symptom Management*, 18: 253–62.

Woollam, C.H. and Jackson, A.O. (1998) Acupuncture in the management of chronic pain, *Anaesthesia*, 53(6): 593–5.

World Health Organization (WHO) (1990) *Cancer Pain Relief and Palliative Care Technical Report Series 8404*. Geneva: WHO.

—— (2007) Case Definitions of HIV for Surveillance and Revised Clinical Staging and Immunological Classification of HIV-related Disease in Adults and Children. Available online at www.who.int/hiv/pub/guidelines/HIVstaging150307.pdf (accessed 30 July 2009).

—— (1986) *Cancer Pain Relief*. Geneva: WHO.

—— (1996) *Cancer Pain Relief: With a Guide to Opioid Availability*, 2nd edn. Geneva: WHO.

—— (2004) *Palliative Care: The Solid Facts*. Geneva: WHO.

Further reading

Motor Neurone Disease Association. Different types of MND (2009) Available online at www.mndassociation.org/life_with_mnd/what_is_mnd/types_of_mnd.html (accessed 28 July 2009).

National Council for Palliative Care. *Supportive and Palliative Care defined*. Available online at www.ncpc.org.uk/palliative_care.html.

Paz, S. and Seymour, J. (2008) *Pain: Theories, Evaluation and Management*, in S. Payne, J. Seymour and C. Ingelton (eds) *Palliative Care Nursing: Principles and Evidence for Practice*. Maidenhead: Open University Press.

Appendix

Gibbs's (1988) model of reflection

Gibbs's model is an uncomplicated approach to reflection with six stages (see Fig. A.1).

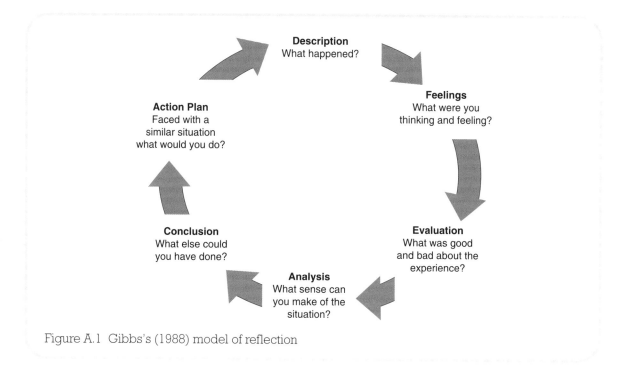

Figure A.1 Gibbs's (1988) model of reflection

Description

Initially describe in detail the incident you have chosen. Think about including the following detail: what you were doing; what were other people doing; where you were; the context of the event; what happened during the event and what part you and others played in the incident. As a result what were the results of people's involvement?

Feelings

What were you thinking and feeling during the incident? Try to link your thoughts and feelings to aspects of the incident. For example, how were you feeling at the start and why did your feelings change? Was it a result of what you were doing or as a result of the individual patient's reactions; or those of other professionals?

Evaluation

Make a judgement about what happened, highlighting the good and not so good aspects of the experience. What went well, and what didn't?

Analysis

During this stage examine each element of the incident and consider why things happened in the way they did. When carrying out this analysis draw on the theory you have studied within the book or further reading to come to an explanation for events. This is an important stage in the reflective process where you are challenging your practice, looking for explanations for why things went well or not and putting this understanding within the context of existing evidence.

Conclusion

This stage is a culmination of the reflection so far. These conclusions are the clarification of your understanding and insight into what happened. You should be identifying elements of your practice which are good and should be continued and ones that need to be reconsidered.

Action plan

The final stage of your reflection asks you to consider what you would do differently next time you encountered a similar situation.

The cycle of reflection is complete until the next time a similar situation occurs where you can reflect once more on the success of the changes you have made. We appreciate that no two situations are identical; nevertheless, reflecting in this way can encourage a thoughtful exploration that develops a critical examination of practice.

Glossary

A

Aβ neurones: (A beta) nerves responding to touch and other forms of non-noxious stimuli, producing a modulating counter-stimulation at the pain gate.

Aδ neurones: (A delta) nerves respond to noxious stimuli, producing fast pain.

action potential: the change in the electrical charge on a neurone cell membrane triggered by a sensory receptor that propagates a nerve impulse.

acupuncture: a complementary therapy that involves inserting fine needles into the body; there is some evidence that this stimulates the sensory nervous system to produce modulation of pain.

adjuvant: non-analgesic drugs that act on the nervous system to modulate pain.

affective: emotional expression.

afferent nerves: neurones that conduct nerve impulses from receptors towards the central nervous system, making up the sensory nervous system.

agonist: a chemical that binds to a receptor and triggers a response.

alkaloids: naturally occurring chemicals derived from plant material that contain nitrogen, and are alkaline in pH; many have strong pharmacological or toxic effects.

allodynia: pain caused by stimuli that are normally non-painful.

amplification: low-level sensory information that is normally not painful provokes pain.

anaesthetic blocks: using a local anaesthetic to block sensation and/or motor in a region of the body in order to perform surgery or provide pain relief.

antagonist: a chemical that binds to a receptor and blocks the action of an agonist.

anti-allodynic: an action that prevents allodynia.

anti-hyperalgesic: an action that prevents hyperalgesia.

anti-pyretic: drugs that reduce fever.

arachnoid mater: the middle of the three meninges, it contains cerebro-spinal fluid between it and the inner pia mater.

arthroplasty: joint replacement surgery.

atelectasis: loss of gas exchange across alveoli due to fluid consolidation.

autonomic nervous system: regulates individual organ function and homeostasis, and for the most part is not subject to voluntary control; it consists of the sympathetic and parasympathetic nervous system.

axon: a part of a neurone in the peripheral nervous system, they appear as long thread-like projections extending from the receptor to the synapse; they are the site of conduction.

B

balanced analgesia: the use of opioids, non-opioids and adjuvants to produce maximum pain relief with minimum dosing of individual drugs with the intention of reducing side-effects; also known as multimodal analgesia.

beneficence: an ethical principle referring to an action that promotes the well-being of others.

biliary colic: visceral pain associated with cholecystitis and gallstones.

biopsychosocial model: a model that explains health in terms of interaction between biological, psychological and social factors.

C

C neurones: nerves responding to noxious stimuli, producing slow pain.

Caesarean section: a surgical procedure in which a low abdominal incision is made into the uterus in order to deliver a baby.

cannabinoid: a group of chemicals found in cannabis and occurring naturally in the nervous system.

catabolism: metabolic process that produces energy from the breakdown of larger molecules into smaller compounds.

catastrophizing: an irrational thought process, believing something is worse than it is.

catecholamine: hormones released by the adrenal glands that trigger the 'fight or flight response' in the sympathetic nervous system.

causalgia: a neuropathic pain disorder now called complex regional pain syndrome type 2.

central pain: a distressing neuropathic pain originating from damage to the central nervous system; for example, after a stroke.

chemoreceptors: respond to chemical stimuli.

chronic pain syndrome: a complex response to chronic pain associated with affective and social as well as biological dysfunction.

clinical governance: the systematic organization of clinical quality adopted by the UK for ensuring quality of care in the NHS.

Co-analgesic: drugs that combine two or more analgesics, usually an opioid with paracetamol, producing a synergistic effect that enhances the effectiveness of each separate analgesic.

cognitive behavioural therapy: a systematic goal-oriented treatment approach that address dysfunctional thoughts, emotions and behaviours.

complex regional pain syndrome (CRPS): neuropathic disorders usually occurring after trauma or tissue damage which involve both the peripheral sensory nervous system and the sympathetic nervous system.

congenital insensitivity to pain with anhydrosis: an extremely rare inherited disorder of the nervous system, mainly affecting noxious stimuli and temperature detection; most sufferers die in early childhood from opportunistic infections and hyperthermia.

counter-stimulation: stimulation of the peripheral nervous system in a non-noxious manner with the aim of modulating pain.

crossover: signals from motor nerves stimulate adjacent nociceptive neurones; seen in diseases which produce demyelination.

D

deafferentation: disruption of sensory conduction due to damage to large diameter neurones, typically caused by trauma, such as brachial plexus avulsion.

delta (δ) receptor: site of action for opioids and endogenous opioid peptides EOP.

dementia: loss of cognitive ability due to abnormal changes in brain structures or function.

demyelination: loss of myelin due to diseases such as multiple sclerosis.

deontological: a moral code that is characterized by adherence to rules or duties.

detrusor muscle: a smooth muscle in the bladder which contracts when urinating.

dorsal horn: the part of the spinal cord where the pain gate is located.

dura mater: the tough outermost membrane of the meninges.

dynorphins: an endogenous opioid peptide.

dysaesthesia: an unpleasant abnormal sensation, stinging, acidic or burning in nature; usually evoked by touch; commonly seen in diabetic neuropathy.

dysphoria: unpleasant or distressing mood.

E

ectopic stimuli: the production of a noxious impulse by a lesion on the axon of a neurone rather than at a nociceptor; locally excitable such lesions can form 'pacemakers' that propagate constant noxious signals.

efferent nerves: neurones that conduct nerve impulses from the central nervous system to muscles and glands in the periphery; the motor nervous system is composed of efferent nerves.

endogenous opioid peptides (EOP): naturally occurring opioid like neurotransmitters that inhibit and modulate pain.

endorphins: an endogenous opioid peptide.

enkephalins: an endogenous opioid peptide.

enteral: pertaining to the digestive tract.

epidural analgesia: the delivery of analgesics into the epidural space; this may be a single dose via an injection or continuous via an infusion through a catheter.

epidural space: the region lying above the dura mater formed from the outer part of the spinal canal.

F

fibromyalgia: a complex painful muscular disorder; symptoms include multiple trigger points, fatigue and low mood.

G

gamma amino butyric acid (GABA): the main inhibitory neurotransmitter, it plays a role regulating excitability and modulates pain.

generator potential: a peripheral nociceptor is stimulated in a graded way, continual stimulation produces a generator potential which when it reaches threshold triggers a volley of action potentials.

glomerular filtration: the process of filtering blood in the kidneys to form urine.

glutamate: the most abundant excitatory neurotransmitter; it acts on the N-methyl-D-aspartic acid (NMDA) receptor to modulate pain.

glycerine trinitrate: a drug used in the treatment of angina and heart failure, it has vasodilating properties; its use is contraindicated in epidural analgesia.

H

height of block: a measurement of the extent of an anaesthetic block.

hyperaesthesia: increased sensitivity to stimuli.

hyperalgesia: excessive sensitivity to unpleasant stimuli which is interpreted as pain; usually seen in neuropathic disorders.

hypercoagulability: an abnormality in clotting that leads to production of thrombosis.

hyperpathia: an abnormal response to nociceptive stimuli that provokes severe pain.

I

iatrogenic: harm, adverse effects or complications arising from medical treatment or advice.

immunosupression: action that inhibits the action of the immune system.

intrathecal: the space under the arachnoid mater in which cerebro-spinal fluid is found (*see spinal*).

ischaemia: restriction in blood supply.

K

kappa (κ) receptor: site of action for opioids and endogenous opioid peptides (EOP).

L

learning disability: in the UK the term 'learning disability' refers to a wide range of disorders; from specific ones related to difficulty in processing information that severely limit a person's ability to learn in a specific skill area to more generalized problems related to impaired cognitive function that may be associated with physical disability as well and that arise during childhood.

limbic region: an area of the brain responsible for emotions, long-term memory and some behaviours; it is involved in affective modulation of pain.

locus of control: a psychological theory describing beliefs and attributes about influences on events in one's life.

M

mechanoreceptors: receptors involved in detection of movement and pressure.

medulla oblongata: the lower portion of the brain stem; it deals with autonomic functions like respiration and temperature control.

minimum effective analgesia concentration: the minimum plasma drug concentration at which analgesia occurs.

modulation: the process in which several opposing neuronal processes regulate noxious signals to produce pain.

morphine-6-beta-glucuronide (M6G): the active metabolite of morphine.

motor block: the action of local anaesthetic on motor nerves stopping conduction along the axon so that central nervous system commands do not reach muscles.

mu (μ) receptor: site of action for opioids and endogenous opioid peptides (EOP), most important receptor for pain modulation.

multidisciplinary: in health this refers to collaborative working in close co-operation between different disciplines leading to mutual and cumulative improvements in assessment, diagnoses, treatment and care for patients.

multimodal analgesia: *see balanced analgesia.*

myelin sheath: a fatty membrane that covers some neurones; its functions include protection and transmission of nerve impulses (myelinated – possessing a myelin sheath, unmyelinated – lacking a myelin sheath).

N

N-methyl-D-aspartic acid receptor (NMDA): the site of action for glutamate.

neuralgia: intense burning or stabbing pain caused by irritation of or damage to a nerve.

neuritis: inflammation to a nerve.

neurokinins: neurotransmitters closely related to substance P and involved in excitation; substance P acts on their receptors.

neuromas: non-malignant tumours, often formed when a nerve is cut; they can be a source of ectopic stimuli and can involve the sympathetic nervous system.

neuropathic: arising from an altered abnormal function, change or damage to a nerve.

neuropeptide: small protein-like neurotransmitters.

neurotransmitters: molecules that allow neurones to communicate with each other at a synapse.

nociceptors: receptors responsible for detecting unpleasant stimuli.

nociceptive: relating to pain that is produced in a normal or healthy nervous system.

Non-steroidal anti-inflammatory drugs (NSAIDs): a group of analgesic drugs that act in the periphery.

nonmaleficence: an ethical principal meaning doing no harm by your actions.

noxious stimulus: unpleasant stimuli that trigger a nociceptive impulse.

O

operator errors: these are mistakes that occur when using technical equipment due to human action.

opioid: a group of analgesics that act on the central nervous system and are either derived from opium or synthesized and act like drugs derived from opium.

opioid resistance pain: pain for which opioids are not effective, as in neuropathic pain.

opium: a naturally occurring chemical substance obtained from opium poppies that contain many compounds, some of which are strong analgesics.

P

pacing: a structured learnt behaviour where activities are controlled in order to avoid excessive rest or overexertion.

paraesthesia: an unpleasant tingling sensation of 'pins and needles'.

paralytic ileus: an absence of peristalsis in the gut, a side-effect of abdominal surgery, general anaesthetics, opioids and some visceral pains.

parenteral: drug administration other than by the mouth or the rectum.

partial agonist: a chemical that binds to a receptor but triggers a less effective response than an agonist.

pathophysiology: the study of changes in normal physiological functions because of disease or abnormality.

patient-controlled analgesia: any system of self-delivery of analgesia, normally refers to the use of a modified 'on demand' intravenous infusion pump.

person-centred: an approach to care that advocates individual choice and empowerment.

phantom pain: a complex neuropathic pain associated with limb amputation or other loss of a body part.

placebo: an inert dummy intervention that is intended to act as a control in medical experiments.

placebo effect: the amount of impact a placebo has on the subjective experience of a patient. In pain this effect is believed to be fairly strong; the effect can be both negative and positive.

polymodal receptors: respond to many stimuli.

prefrontal cortex: the anterior part of the cerebral cortex; it is where pain is perceived and cognitive processes integrate.

preloading: in epidural management, preloading with intravenous fluid compensates for the vasodilating effects of local anaesthetic and therefore maintains a normal blood pressure.

primary hyperalgesia: increased excitability of peripheral nociceptors mainly due to tissue damage and inflammation.

pro-drug: a pharmacological substance that is converted to an active drug by metabolic processes.

prophylactic: protecting against infection or disease.

proprioception: detection of signals that locate different parts of the body and relate them to each other.

proprioreceptors: receptors involved in proprioception.

pruritus: intense itching.

R

rank scoring: a method of measuring differences between two points that does not use equal intervals between scores. In a verbal rating scale the difference between moderate and severe pain is not the same as the difference between no pain and mild pain.

receptors: the part of the neurone responsible for detecting stimuli, located at the distal end of the neurone.

reflex arc: a spontaneous motor response to intense nociception that removes the damaged site away from the cause of injury; also known as a spinal cord reflex.

reflex sympathetic dystrophy: a neuropathic disorder now called complex regional pain syndrome type 1.

reticular formation: an area of the brain stem,

involved in pain modulation and is believed to be a location for descending analgesic pathways.

rubefacient: a topical substance that produces redness of the skin when rubbed on.

S

sensory block: the action of local anaesthetic on sensory nerves stopping conduction along the axon so that peripheral stimuli do not reach the central nervous system.

serotonin: an inhibitory pain neurotransmitter involved in mood and sleep; in the periphery it is released through inflammatory processes and stimulates nociceptors.

slow pain: noxious stimuli carried by C neurones characterized by dull, longer-lasting, aching pain.

somatic: relating to or affecting the body; in pain it particularly refers to muscles, skin and bones.

sphincter of Oddi: a muscular valve that controls the flow of digestive juices from the gall bladder and pancreas into the small intestine.

spinal: an injection into the intrathecal space.

spinal cord reflex: *see reflex arc.*

spinal nerves: pairs of nerves that exit the spinal cord at each vertebral level; they carry sensory and motor information to a specific zone of the body.

spinothalamic tract: a sensory pathway that ascends the spinal cord to the thalamus and carries information about pain and temperature.

subdural: under the dura mater.

substance P: an excitatory neuropeptide.

summation: intense repeated stimuli produce pain that lasts for longer than each stimulus.

surgical stress response: the pathophysiological impact of surgery on multiple organ systems.

sympathetic nervous system: part of the autonomic nervous system, it acts to maintain the body in a state of homeostasis and is involved in mobilizing body responses at times of stress.

sympathetically maintained pains: pains which are exacerbated or caused by abnormal actions of the sympathetic nervous system (*see complex regional pain syndrome* (CRPS)).

sympathectomy: the removal or destruction of parts of the sympathetic nervous system by surgery or chemical means. This reduces sympathetic action and can be a treatment for sympathetically maintained pains.

T

thalamus: situated between the brain stem and the cortex, the thalamus has many functions; in pain it is a site of modulation.

thermoreceptors: receptors involved in temperature detection.

thoracotomy: a surgical procedure involving an incision into the chest wall.

threshold: the minimum state of excitation at which a stimulus will trigger a receptor to produce an action potential.

tolerance: the degree of pain a person can experience before it becomes unbearable; unlike pain threshold, it is affected by biopsychosocial factors and varies greatly between people.

total pain experience: the unique individual response to pain arising from an interaction between physiological, social and psychological processes; some commentators also include spiritual aspects in this concept.

transcutaneous electrical nerve stimulation (TENS): a therapeutic technique believed to modulate pain through counter-stimulation.

transduction: the process of converting a stimulus from one form to another, at a receptor or synapse, which is then transmitted along an axon.

trigeminal neuralgia: a neuropathic pain involving the fifth cranial nerve affecting the face and jaw.

trigger point: a locally occurring well-defined tense spot in muscle that can be felt as a lump on palpation and produces a strong pain response that radiates along the length of the muscle when firm pressure is applied.

trycyclic antidepressant: a group of drugs with a similar three-ringed molecular formula, originally developed in the 1950s for treating mood disorders: They also act as an adjuvant in the central nervous system to modulate pain.

U

utilitarianism: a moral code that is characterized by balancing possible outcomes and settling on the one that produces the greater happiness for all concerned.

V

visceral: relating to or affecting the internal organs.

vasodilatation: widening of the blood vessels as a

consequence of relaxation of smooth muscles in vessel walls.

ventral nuclei: region of the thalamus associated with pain transmission and modulation.

W

wind-up: repeated intense stimulation of nociceptors produces changes in neurotransmitter activity in the dorsal horn of the spinal cord. These changes lead to hyperalgesia and allodynia.

Index

Locators shown in *italics* refer to case studies, figures and tables.

Abbey, J., 171
abnormal central processing
    role in pain experience, 51
absorption
    as variable in drug effectiveness, 89–90
    rate of as factor in drug delivery route, 94
actions, drug
    duration of, 96–9, *97, 98, 99*
    effectiveness of, 89–91, *91*
    mechanisms for, 90
    see also delivery, drugs
activity, physical
    role in palliative pain management, 179–80
'activity cycling'
    as measure of pain scores, 157, *157*
acupuncture
    role in palliative pain management, 180
acute pain
    characteristics and purpose of person-centred management,
        131–2, *132*
    ensuring adherence to care, 134–6
    ethical considerations of management, 133–4, *133*
    implications of surgical stress responses to, 127–8, *127*
    management plans for, 136–40, *137, 140*
    physical effects of unmanaged, 126–7, *126*
    see also plans, pain management
Acute Pain Service (APS), 111–13
adaptation, patient
    chronic pain, 146–7, *147*
    see also perceptions, patient
    see also influences eg depression
administration, drugs *see* delivery, drugs
adults
    pain assessment and management tools for, 70–73, *71, 73*
AIDS and HIV
    causes of pain in, 168–9, *168*
Alimi, D., 180
amplification
    as element of neuropathic pain, 49–51, *50*
anaesthesia, local
    role in palliative pain management, 178–9
    use in management of pain, 106
analgesia
    case study of moral dilemmas surrounding, 21, *21*
    duration of action, 96–9, *97, 98, 99*
    factors determining choice, 88–9
    guidelines for use in palliative care, 177–80, *177, 178, 179*
    routes of administration, 93–5
    salience of balancing of, 128

    see also drug names and types eg anti-convulsants; anti-
        depressants; corticosteroids; cannabinoids; capsaicin; NSAIDs;
        opiods; paracetamol
    see also influences on effectiveness eg concentration, plasma
    see also type eg anaesthesia, local; epidurals; patient-controlled
        analgesia
anger, patient
    coping strategies in chronic pain, 157
anti-convulsants
    use in management of pain, 105
anti-depressants
    use in management of pain, 105
anxiety and fear, patient
    as influence on pain experience and assessment, 67–8, *67*
    avoidance strategies for chronic pain, 154–7, *154, 155, 156*
    coping strategies in chronic pain, 157
    influence on pain responses, 172
Apfelbaum, J., 126
appraisal, cognitive
    influence on pain responses, 172
APS (Acute Pain Service), 111–13
Arkes, H., 135, 136
aromatherapy
    role in palliative pain management, 180
assessment, pain
    attitudes exhibited by healthcare staff to, 174–5
    definition, purpose and frequency, 62, 68–70, *69*
    effectiveness and importance in care planning, 63, 73, 169–70
    influence of patient anxiety and fear on, 67–8, *67*
    problems associated with process, 63–4, *64*
    see also management, pain; tools, pain assessment and
        management
    see also specific types and clientele eg children; chronic pain;
        palliative pain
Association of Anaesthetists of Great Britain and Ireland, 110, 112
Audit Commission, 67–9, 110
autonomy
    principles assisting healthcare decisions, 28–30, *29, 30*

Beebe, A., 6, 7, 9
Beech, M., 180
behaviours, moral
    effects of illness on, 20–22
behaviours, patient
    chronic pain coping, 154–7, *154, 155, 156*
    see also perceptions, patient
beneficence
    as bioethical principle assisting healthcare, 30–31
Bentham, J., 25

bioethics and ethics *see* ethics and bioethics
biomedicine
    model of pain experience, 10–12
biopsychosocial
    model of pain experience, 12–16, *13, 15*
    role in communication of pain experience, 37–8
Bogduk, N., 56
Bond, M., 172
Bonica, J., 67, 110
Boyle, P., 172
brain
    anatomy and role in pain experiences, 46–8, *47*
Brief Pain Inventory (BPI), 77, 78, *79–80, 79, 80–81*, 171
Breitbart, W., 168, 177–8
Breivik, H., 144–6, *147*, 149
British Pain Society, 150
Brockopp, D., 65

cancer
    approaches to pain management, 175–6, *176*
    causes of pain in, 165–6
Cancer research UK, 165
cannabinoids
    use in management of pain, 106
capability, patient
    salience in pain risk management, 116–17, *116, 117*
    see also intellect, patient; knowledge, patient; understanding,
        patient
capsaicin
    use in management of pain, 106
cardiovascular system
    implications of acute pain on response of, 127, *127*
care, end of life *see* palliative care
Carr, E., 64, 65, 67
Carter, B., 4
case studies
    assessment of chronic pain, *76*
    pain management, 25–8, *26, 113, 116, 117, 132*
    pain medication, 21, *21*
    patient consent, 32–3, *33*
    patient intellectual capability in pain management, *117*
    unmanaged acute pain, *126*
CBT (cognitive behavioural therapy), 179–80
'central pain', 51–2
central processing, normal
    role in pain experience, 51
Challenge of Pain, The (Melzack), 40
charts, rating
    as pain assessment tool, 70–73, *71, 73*
chemotherapy
    role in palliative pain management, 178
children
    chronic pain assessment of, 81–2
    pain assessment and management tools, 73–5, *74, 75*
choice, patient
    salience in pain risk management, 116
    see also consent, patient; knowledge, patient
chronic pain
    assessment of in children, 81–2
    assessment types, 77–8
    case study of assessment of, *76*
    definition and characteristics, 77, 144–6, *145*

history and organisation of management of, 110–11, *110,*
    149–54, *153*
    impact on family and friends of sufferer with, 148
    patient perceptions and coping behaviours, 75–7, *76*, 154–7, *154,*
        155, 156
    psychosocial factors influencing experience, 171–4
    role of pain assessment tools, 78–81, *79–80*
    salience of pain history in assessment of, 78
    see also adaptation, patient; perceptions, patient; plans, pain
        management
Chronic Pain Syndrome (CPS), 146–9, *147*
Chumbley, G., 114
Cicala, R., 180
classifications
    of pain, 4–9
    see also models and theories
Clinical Standards Advisory Group (CSAG), 64, 67
codeine, 104
cognition
    influence on pain responses, 172
cognitive behavioural therapy (CBT), 179–80
Coll, A-M., 72
communication, pain
    intrapersonal perspective, 37–9, 40–42, *39, 41, 43, 44–5*
    models and theories of, 39–40, 52–3, *53, 55*
    role in communication of pain, 43–4, *45, 46*
    role of action potentials, 43–4
    role of brain, 46–8, *47*
    role of cutaneous and visceral receptors, 42–3, *43*
    role of sensory nerves, 44
    see also experiences and responses, pain; neurotransmitters and
        neurotransmission
    see also elements eg detection; modulation; perception
    see also tools eg nerves, sensory; neurotransmitters and
        neurotransmission; receptors, cutaneous and visceral
Complex Regional Pain Syndrome (CRPS), 51
complications
    management of in pain control, 115–19, *116, 117, 118*
    see also influencing factors eg staff, healthcare
concentration, plasma
    influence of drug action duration, 96–9, *97, 98, 99*
    relationship with drug target site, 95–6, *95*
conditions, life limiting
    definition and characteristics, 164–5, *165*
    definitions of pain in, 165
    psychosocial factors influencing experience of, 171–4
    see also specific eg cancer; HIV and AIDS; Multiple Sclerosis
    see also treatments eg assessment, pain
consent, patient
    case study of, 32–3, *33*
    see also choice, patient; knowledge, patient
control, loss of
    as influence on pain experience and assessment, 67–8
control, patient
    influence on pain responses, 172
coping, patient
    influence on pain responses, 172–3
Copp, L., 172–3
cortex, 47–8
corticosteroids
    use in management of pain, 105
Cousins, M., 171

CPS (Chronic Pain Syndrome), 146–9, *147*
Craig, K., 52, 55
CRPS (Complex Regional Pain Syndrome), 51
culture
    influence on pain responses, 171–2

Davey, B., 33
Davies, H., 73
Deep, P., 12–13
delivery, drugs
    pharmacological compartmental model of, 91–3, *92, 93*
    routes of administration, 93–5
    salience of plasma concentration on target site, 95–6, *95*
    see also outcomes eg actions, drug
deontology, 23–5
dependence
    as feature of opioids, 105
depression
    coping strategies in chronic pain, 157
    response to chronic pain, 147–8
detection
    role in communication of pain, 42, *43*
diamorphine, 103
diaries, patient
    as pain assessment tool, 81
    as pain management tool, *156*
distribution
    as variable in drug effectiveness, 90
dosing, drug repeat, 96–9, *97, 98, 99*
drugs, pain management
    barriers to successful use, 176
    case study of, 21, *21*
    effectiveness of, 89–91, *91*
    risks and side effects, 118–19
    see also actions, drug; delivery, drugs
    see also care setting eg palliative care
    see also specific and types eg anaesthesia, local; analgesia; anti-convulsants; anti-depressants; cannabinoids; opiods
Dunn, V., 62, 64
duties, healthcare staff
    role in pain management, 28
    see also consent, patient

education, patient
    influence of observational on pain responses, 172
    salience and use in pain management, 113–15, *113*
    see also knowledge, patient
effectiveness, drug
    absorption as variable of, 89–90
    distribution as variable of, 90
    metabolism as variable of, 90–91
endocrinology
    role in palliative pain management, 178
Engel, G., 12
epidurals
    complications and risks, 119
equivalence
    factor in drug delivery route, 94–5
ethics and bioethics
    as consideration in person-centred pain management, 133–4, *133*
    role in deciding healthcare issues, 28–33, *29, 30, 33*

usefulness in organising pain management, 33–4
    see also type eg deontology; utilitarianism
Europe
    prevalence of chronic pain in, 144–6, *145*
experiences and responses, pain
    duration and function, 5–7
    influences on, 53–5, 67–8, 171–3
    socio-communication model of, 52–3, *53, 55*, 55–8
    see also communication, pain
extroversion, patient
    influence on pain responses, 172

family and friends
    impact of chronic pain sufferer on well-being of, 148
Faull, C., 165
fear and anxiety, patient *see* anxiety and fear, patient
fentanyl, 104
Fordham, M., 62, 64
formation, reticular, 46–7
friends and family
    impact of chronic pain sufferer on well-being of, 148

Garbez, R., 134
gastrointestinal system
    implications of acute pain on response of, 127–8, *127*
gate control theory of pain, 40
gates, pain
    as site for modulation of pain, 44–6
Gibbs, G., 185–6, *185*
Gould, T., 68, 73
Graham, J., 157
Gwatkin, D., 34

Harmer, M., 73, 130
healthcare
    bioethical principles assisting, 28–33, *29, 30, 33*
    see also staff, healthcare
Heavner, J., 134
heroin, 103
Herring, J., 27
HIV and AIDS
    causes of pain in, 168–9, *168*
hyperalgesia
    role in communication of pain, 43, 45

IASP (International Association for the Study of Pain), 9, 56, 77, *154*
Idvall, E., 120–21
illness
    effects of on moral behaviours, 20–22
imagery, guided
    role in palliative pain management, 180
immobilization
    role in palliative pain management, 180–81
impulses abnormal
    as element of neuropathic pain, 49, *50*
inflammation
    salience in communication of pain, 43
intellect, patient
    salience in pain risk management, 117–18, *117*
    see also capability, patient; knowledge, patient; understanding, patient

International Association for the Study of Pain (IASP), 9, 56, 77, *154*
introversion, patient
  influence on pain responses, 172

Jackson, A., 180
Jensen, M., 71, 73
journals, patient
  as pain assessment tool, 81
justice
  principle assisting healthcare decisions, 31–3, *33*

Kant, I., 23–5
Karoly, P., 71, 73
Kastanias, P., 114
Kaye, P., 165
knowledge, patient
  salience in pain management, 114–15
  see also capability, patient; intellect, patient; understanding, patient

learning, patient
  influence of observational on pain responses, 172
  salience and use in pain management, 113–15, *113*
  see also knowledge, patient
lipids, solubility of
  factor in drug delivery route, 94
Lisson, E., 29
Littlejohn, C., 118
Loeser, J., 6, 7, 56

McCaffrey, M., 6, 7, 9
McCracken, L., 155
McGill Pain Questionnaire (MPQ), 78, 79–80, *80–81*, 171
McGrath, P., 15
McIntyre, P., 130, 133
Main, C., 12
management, pain
  approaches, principles and strategies, 20, 63–8, *65, 67*
  case studies of, 25–8, *26, 113*
  history, organisation and purpose, 110–11, *110*
  need for staff support and development, 120–21, *120*
  salience of pain in developing principles for, 33–4, *34*
  salience of patient knowledge and education, 113–15, *113*
  salience of risk management, 115–19, *116, 117, 118*
  see also assessment, pain; plans, pain management; tools, pain assessment and management
  see also elements eg drugs, pain management; immobilization; rehabilitation
  see also influences eg duties, healthcare staff; ethics and bioethics; rights, patient
  see also particular services eg acute pain service; palliative care
  see also specific clientele and pain types eg acute pain, children; chronic pain; palliative pain
management, risk
  salience in pain management, 115–19, *116, 117, 118*
  see also influencing factors eg staff, healthcare
massage
  role in palliative pain management, 180
medication, pain management see drugs, pain management
meditation
  role in palliative pain management, 180

Melzack, R., 2, 40, 45, 65, 78
Memorial Pain Assessment Card (MPAC), 171
Merskey, H., 56
metabolism, patient
  as variable in drug effectiveness, 90–91
methadone, 104
Mintzer, B., 133
modelling
  influence on pain responses, 172
  see also scores, modelling
models and theories
  communication of pain experience, 39–40
  compartmental model of pharmacokinetics, 91–3, *92, 93*
  nature of pain, 40–42, *41*
  pain experience, 10–16, *13, 15*
  reflective practice, 185–6, *185*
  sociocommunication model of pain responses, 52–3, *53, 55–8*
modulation
  role in communication of pain, 42, *43*
  see also sites eg gates, pain
morals and morality
  as benchmark for deciding pain responses, 22–3
  principles of, 20
  see also behaviours, moral; ethics and bioethics
MPAC (Memorial Pain Assessment Card), 171
MPQ (McGill Pain Questionnaire), 78, 79–80, *80–81*, 171
Multiple Sclerosis (MS)
  causes of pain in, 166–8, *166, 167*
Multiple Sclerosis Society, 166

National Council for Hospice and Specialist Palliative Care Services (NCHSPCS), 163
National Council for Palliative Care, 181
National Health and Medical Research Council (NHMRC), 67
National Institute for Health and Clinical Excellence (NICE), 163–4, 181
NCHSPCS (National Council for Hospice and Specialist Palliative Care Services), 163
nerves, sensory
  role in transmission of pain, 44
neuropathic pain, 48–52, *49, 50*
neuroticism
  influence on pain responses, 172
neurotransmitters and neurotransmission
  role in communication of pain, 45, *46*
NHMRC (National Health and Medical Research Council), 67
NICE (National Institute for Health and Clinical Excellence), 163–4, 181
nociceptive pain
  characteristics, 40–42, *41, 50, 52*
  see also elements eg gate, pain
  see also influences eg brain
nonmaleficence
  as bioethical principle assisting healthcare, 31
NSAIDs, 99–101, *100*
Numerical Rating Scale (NRS), 72–3, *73*

observation
  influence of on pain responses, 172
  see also knowledge, patient
opioids, 101–5, *103*

pain
  definitions, experiences and responses to, 2–4, *3*, 22–3,
    55–7
  factors influencing experience and consequences of, 171–4
  models and classifications of, 4–16, *5*, *13*, *15*
  nature of, 37–42, *39*, *41*, 48–52, *49*, *50*
  see also assessment, pain; communication, pain; management,
    pain
  see also types and diseases eg acute pain; AIDS and HIV;
    capsaicin; chronic pain; Multiple Sclerosis; palliative pain
painkillers *see* analgesia
pains, sympathetically maintained (SMPs), 51
palliative care
  definition and characteristics, 162–3, *162–3*
  see also conditions, life limiting; supportive care; terminal care
  see also elements eg assessment, pain; management, pain
palliative pain
  guidelines for analgesia use in, 177–80, *177*, *178*, *179*
  history, organisation and purpose of care for, 111
  pharmacological and non-pharmacological in management of,
    175
  role of immobilization in management of, 180–81
  role of pain assessment tools, 170–71
  role of physical activity in management of, 179–80
  role of radiotherapy in management of, 178
  role of rehabilitation in management of, 181
  significance and role of pain assessment, 169–70
paracetamol, 101
Parbrook, G., 172
Parsons, S., 144, 145
partners
  impact of chronic pain on well-being of, 148
Patel, J., 147
pathophysiology
  of pain experience, 7
Patient-Controlled Analgesia (PCA)
  definition and characteristics, 128–9
  principles of application, 129–31, *129*, *130*
Payne, S., 161
perceptions, patient
  chronic pain management, 150–54, *153*
  see also behaviours, patient
pethidine, 104
'phantom pain', 52
pharmacokinetics
  compartmental model of, 91–3, *92*, *93*
Phillips, C., 33
plans, pain management
  characteristics and evaluation of chronic, 149–54, *153*
  characteristics, evaluation in acute, 138–40, *140*
  problems with goals and outcomes in acute, 136–8, *137*
plasma
  salience on drug delivery targets site, 95–6, *95*
Popay, J., 33
potentials, action
  role in transmission of pain, 43–4
Powell, B., 64
practice, reflective
  theoretical model of, 185–6, *185*
principles (concept)
  characteristics and definition in pain management, 20
  see also subject eg ethics and bioethics; morals and morality

processing, abnormal central
  role in pain experience, 51
psychology
  role in palliative pain management, 179–80

Quality Adjusted Life Year (QALY), 27–8
questionnaires
  as pain assessment tool, 78–81, *80–1*, 171

radiotherapy
  role in palliative pain management, 178
Raising the Standard (RCA), 68
Rathmel, J., 133
rating, pain assessment
  use of scales as tools, 70–75, *71*, *73*, *74*, *75*
receptors, cutaneous and visceral
  role in transmission and distribution of pain, 42–3, *43*
reflection
  theoretical model of, 185–6, *185*
reflexology
  role in palliative pain management, 180
Reflex Sympathetic Dystrophy, 51
rehabilitation
  role in palliative pain management, 181
relaxation
  role in palliative pain management, 180
respiration
  implications of acute pain on response of, 127, *127*
responses and experiences, pain
  duration and function, 5–7
  influences on, 53–5, 67–8, 171–3
  moral beliefs as benchmark for deciding, 22–3
  socio-communication model of, 52–3, *53*, 55–8
  see also communication, pain
rights, patient
  role in pain management, 28
  see also choice, patient; consent, patient
risks
  management of in pain control, 115–19, *116*, *117*, *118*
  see also influencing factors eg staff, healthcare
Royal College of Anaesthetists, 68, 69, 111
Royal College of General Practitioners, 150
Royal College of Surgeons, 64, 66, 111

Salmon, P., 67
Samuel, V., 155
Saunders, C., 110
scales, measurement
  as pain assessment tool, 70–75, *71*, *73*, *74*, *75*
  as pain management tool, 154–7, *154*, *155*, *156*, *157*
Schafheutle, E., 120
Schneider, 148
Schofield, P., 171
scores, modelling
  as pain assessment tool, 70–75, *71*, *73*, *74*, *75*
  as pain management tool, 154–7, *154*, *155*, *156*, *157*
Scottish Intercollegiate Guidelines Network (SIGN), 177
sensitization
  as element of neuropathic pain, 48–9, *49*
Short form 36 Health Survey (SF-36), 80–81, *79*
Short form Brief Pain Inventory (BPI), 80–81, *79*, *81*
Short form McGill Pain Questionnaire, *79*

sickness
    effects of on moral behaviours, 20–22
SIGN (Scottish Intercollegiate Guidelines Network), 177
Singh, M., 147
Smith, 57
SMPs (Sympathetically Maintained Pains), 51
solubility, lipid
    factor in drug delivery route, 94
Spanswick, C., 12
speed, drug absorption
    factor in drug delivery route, 94
spouses
    impact of chronic pain sufferer on well-being of, 148
staff, healthcare
    attitudes to pain assessment, 174–5
    need for support in developing pain management, 120–21, *120*
    see also duties, healthcare staff
Stein, J., 66
Sternbach, R., 171
Stewart, M., 131
strategies, pain management *see* management, pain
stress, surgical
    implication of responses on acute pain, 127–8, *127*
subjectivism, patient
    as pain assessment tool, 70–71
suitability, patient
    salience in pain risk management, 115–16
    see also influences eg capability, patient; intellect, patient; understanding, patient
supportive care
    definition and characteristics, 163–4, *162–3*
    see also elements eg management, pain
surgery
    role in palliative pain management, 178
Sympathetically Maintained Pains (SMPs), 51
system, respiratory
    implications of acute pain on response of, 127, *127*

tables, measurement
    as pain assessment tool, 70–75, *71, 73, 74, 75*
    as pain management tool, 154–7, *154, 155, 156, 157*
techniques, pain management *see* management, pain
TENS (Transcutaneous Electrical Nerve Stimulation)
    role in palliative pain management, 180
terminal care
    definition and characteristics, 164, *162–3*
    see also palliative care; supportive care
    see also elements eg assessment, pain; management, pain
thalamus, 47, *47*
theories and models *see* models and theories
therapies, complementary
    role in palliative pain management, 180
therapy, endocrine
    role in palliative pain management, 178
Thomas, V., 171

tolerance
    as feature of opioids, 104–5
tools, pain assessment and management
    for chronic pain, 78–81, *79–80*
    for pain in adults, 70–73, *71, 73*
    for pain in children, 73–5, *74, 75*
    role in palliative care, 170–71
    see also scales, measurement
    see also specific eg diaries, patient; journals, patient
Torgerson, W., 78–9
Transcutaneous Electrical Nerve Stimulation (TENS)
    role in palliative pain management, 180
transmission, pain *see* communication, pain
treatment, pain *see* management, pain
Trim, J., 119–21
Tursky, 171
Twycross, R., 165, 176

understanding, patient
    salience in pain management, 113–14, *113*
    see also capability, patient; intellect, patient; knowledge, patient
United Kingdom
    prevalence of chronic pain in, 144–6, *145*
utilitarianism
    bioethical characteristics, 25
    case study of as approach to pain management, 25–8, *26*

verbal rating scales (VRS)
    as pain assessment tool, 71–2, *71*
Verbunt, J., 78
visual analogue scales (VAS)
    as pain assessment tool, 72, *73*

Walker, M., 16
Wall, P., 40, 45, 65, 151–2
Warfield, C., 66
wellbeing, family
    impact of chronic pain suffering on, 148
Wheatley, R., 115–16
White, A., 4
Wilcock A., 165, 176
Williams, A., 34
Williams, B., 112, 115–16
withdrawal
    as feature of opioids, 105
Wisconsin Brief Pain Inventory (BPI), 77, 78, 79–80, *80–81*
Wong-Baker Faces Pain Rating Scale, 74, *74*
Woof, R., 165
Woollam, C., 180
workers, healthcare
    attitudes to pain assessment, 174–5
    need for support in developing pain management, 120–21, *120*
    see also duties, healthcare staff
World Health Organisation, 163, 164, 166, *168*, 175, *176*, 177–80, *177, 178, 179*

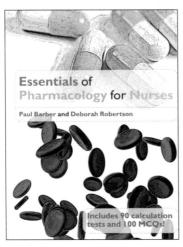

ESSENTIALS OF PHARMACOLOGY FOR NURSES

Paul Barber and Deborah Robertson

9780335234042 (Paperback)
2009

eBook also available

This accessible book introduces pharmacology and calculations in a friendly, informative way. The book focuses on the pharmacology knowledge needed at pre-registration level and does not assume previous knowledge of pharmacology, or a level of confidence with maths and drugs calculations.

Key features:

- Calculation sections containing 90 calculations to help perfect calculation skills
- Clinical tip boxes linking pharmacology to the role of the nurse
- Patient scenarios from a range of different clinical settings, demonstrating pharmacology in clinical settings

www.openup.co.uk

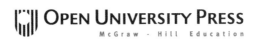
OPEN UNIVERSITY PRESS
McGraw - Hill Education

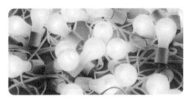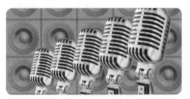
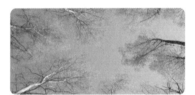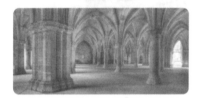
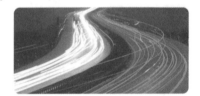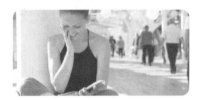
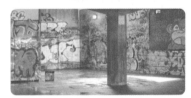
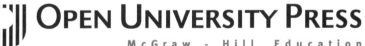